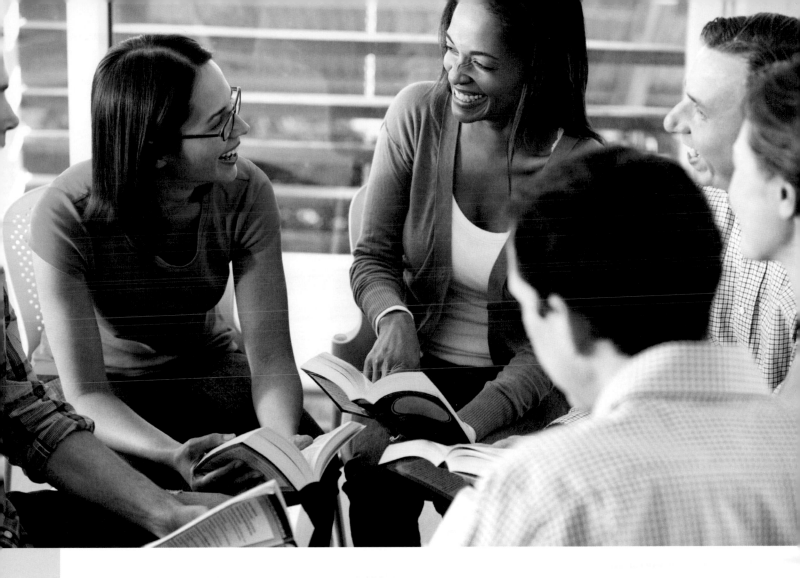

Want to join a Living Wellness Growth Group?

Find a group near you!

Go to AshleyDarkenwald.com to sign up and get more information.

If you don't see a group in your area,
consider becoming a certified Living Wellness Facilitator and
give encouragement to others
seeking health and wellness in your area.

PRAISE FOR
Living Wellness for Growth Groups

As a former fitness professional, I so appreciate a comprehensive approach to health (mind, body, spirit). Ashley Darkenwald has created a health resource that's easy to understand, absolutely attainable, and applicable to our everyday lives. If you're in need of a fresh start or you have questions about nutrition, exercise, or even establishing new healthy habits, take the time to work your way through the pages of this book. You'll be glad you did.

—SUSIE LARSON, talk radio host, national speaker, author of *Your Powerful Prayers*

As a provider of health care for women, I encourage my patients to read *Living Wellness for Growth Groups*. The second edition further promotes insightful means of maintaining control of one's overall health. The information on osteoporosis and its prevention is accurate and thorough. A "must-read" for one who seeks a lifestyle of balance and wellness!

—DR. DANIEL T. CHOW, MD

Ashley passionately, effectively, and caringly reminds us that God is with us every step of the way on our journey through life, including the journey to better health. She shows that He cares about our physical health, just as our spiritual health; that we were created for more than mediocrity, pain, and being overweight. Then she helps find the way to the abundance that our dear Father has promised by stepping through goal setting, providing information to accomplish those goals, and encouraging us to trust God every step of the way. This is a very thoughtful, healing book and I know you will love it!

—KELLEY SUGGS, CHES (certified health education specialist) and natural health practitioner

Great book! *Living Wellness for Growth Groups* will give you many ideas and great motivation to get healthy from the inside out. I am sure you will pick up several ideas from this book, even if you are a well-seasoned reader in the areas of health and weight loss. The ideas are attractively presented with pictures, charts, and graphs, making it easy and interesting to read. Read it and see if your health doesn't improve! Excellent work, Ashley Darkenwald.

—Dr. Mark Virkler, president of Christian Leadership University

I have enjoyed the way this book has been written, especially the easy-to-understand nutritional information. The details and pictures of the exercises will help individuals and participants in growth groups burn fat and get stronger. I love the devotions at the end of the chapter and I look forward to reading the devotional! In the Southeast Appalachian of Kentucky, 80 percent of my patients are overweight or obese with three or more complications of this condition, such as diabetes, hypertension, hyperlipidemia, cardiovascular disease, etc. It saddens me that many of my patients are in their early 40's. The majority do not know what healthy eating means. *Living Wellness for Growth Groups* will help them understand more than a short visit to the clinic.

—SYLVIA Y. SOUTHWORTH, PA-C

I am pleased to see a holistic approach in *Living Wellness for Growth Groups* that includes nutrition, wellness, exercise, and a faith-based foundation. Such a combination breathes fuel for the mind, body, and soul.

—KRISTINE HAERTL, PhD, OTR/L, FAOTA, author, professor

In a world that shifts like sand, *Living Wellness for Growth Groups* is something to stand on. Ashley Darkenwald speaks to your body, mind, and spirit. And she introduces you to the power of community! A small group of companions is waiting to travel with you and cheer you on toward greater health. So open these pages, be inspired, and watch what God can do!

—BJORN DIXON, MDiv, pastor, the WHY Church in Elk River, Minnesota

I thoroughly enjoyed reading *Living Wellness for Growth Groups*. I highly recommend it to those desiring to make a minor or major change in their wellness. *Living Wellness for Growth Groups* is well-researched, balanced, simple to understand, and a great tool for individuals and families who are serious about improving their health.

—CAROLE JOY SEID, MA in education, speaker and consultant for home educators

There are very few readings that will inspire, energize, and transform one's mind-set like what Ashley Darkenwald has put together in *Living Wellness for Growth Groups*. We all need inspiration and ways to reach heights that are often difficult to achieve. Ashley has designed a way to be successful for all walks of life. To the professional with time restraints and the person looking for consistent motivation—commit to reading *Living Wellness for Growth Groups* a day or two every week and you will find a path of positive opportunities for a lifetime.
This is a multiple, MUST-read journey!

—STEVE FESSLER, PGA professional

What *Living Wellness for Growth Groups* Participants Are Saying

I never realized there was a spiritual component to my health. I now view my body as a temple of God. I'm so much more careful about what I eat, and it doesn't feel like punishment; it feels like freedom.
—Linda E.

I loved when you were talking about how what we eat becomes a part of us. I think that is so profound and is very helpful in framing a new belief system around food.
—Tony D.

Thank you, Ashley and team, for designing a wellness program from the heart! The first night's group meeting was a blast! I experienced laughter, fellowship, wisdom, heart, and a safe place to share my thoughts. Our group discovered real and informative information that just makes you want to make a difference in your life. There was no judgment, no condemnation. The meeting was about learning to have a love for my health and wellness! Invest the time in yourself! Be your best self with the love and dedication of Ashley and her team. Your journey will be simply inwardly and outwardly life-changing!
–Pamela P.

I started eating mindfully for the first time in my life. It's the only thing I have really done so far in our group. I am feeling better, I have lost weight, and for the first time, weight loss hasn't been painful.

—Fred B.

I'm still struggling to stay consistent with my portion sizes. I have one good week and one bad week. But I know that I will see this group each week and become stronger and more encouraged to make better decisions. I can do this. Thank you.

—Dennis J.

I was so excited to start the week knowing we had such healthy choices waiting for us! Today was a success, and I worked out at 5:00 a.m.! Just had to share my mini celebration with you. :) Thank you for all you do to guide me, and the group, on this journey to wellness!

You are appreciated.

–Kim S.

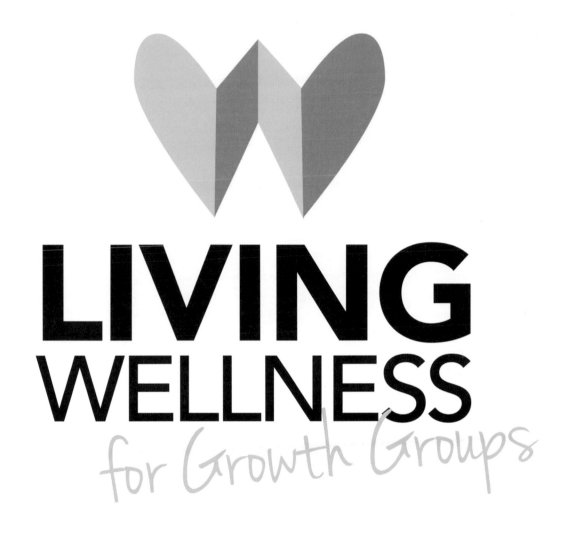

LIVING
WELLNESS
for Growth Groups

Ashley Darkenwald, MS, CPT, PES

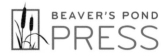
BEAVER'S POND
PRESS

ISBN 13: 978-1-59298-743-6

Library of Congress Catalog Number: 2016920947

Printed in the United States of America

First Printing: 2017

21 20 19 18 17   5 4 3 2 1

Cover design by James Monroe Design, LLC.
Interior design by Dan Pitts.

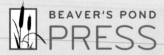

BEAVER'S POND
PRESS

Beaver's Pond Press, Inc.
7108 Ohms Lane
Edina, MN 55439-2129
(952) 829-8818

www.BeaversPondPress.com

To order, visit www.AshleyDarkenwald.com or www.ItascaBooks.com
or call (800) 901-3480. Reseller discounts available.

DEDICATION

Dad, you always taught me to train for life rather than simply study to pass the test. You always told me that you're proud of me. You are the first person I call when I think I'm in a crisis. You listen to me when I'm full of self-pity, and then you swiftly encourage me to get out of the *pit*! Like King David, you are a man after God's own heart. I respect you, and I love you. Thank you for always being yourself and always encouraging me to be me! This book is dedicated to you.

CONTENTS

Week 3

Week 4

Week 5

Week 6

Week 7

Week 8: Finishing Well & Breaking through the Health Barrier . . 218

FOREWORD

You have picked up a very special book, a rare gem. Let me tell you about it.

I am the pastor of a church that calls a large fitness center our home. Every day at the office, I see people come in and out the doors to attend a class, or run on a treadmill, or swim in the pool, or lift weights. It is a steady stream of names and faces from early in the morning until late at night! Fitness is of ever-increasing importance in our culture, especially as we battle back against the forces of obesity, diabetes, and heart disease—to name a few. There is a growing fitness movement across our communities, and it is exciting to see!

But there is something much subtler that has caught my eye. Of all the people pursuing greater fitness, some seem to attain something more—something deeper, something more life-changing than just a trimmer waistline. Rather than just greater fitness, some people find true health.

Ashley Darkenwald knows about finding true health. She knows about the deeper, life-changing aspects of fitness and wellness. And in this book she will take you there.

But not just Ashley. No, you must have other companions at your side for this kind of journey! In *Living Wellness for Growth Groups* you will experience one of the key ingredients for making lasting change in your life: *other people*! Remember all those people streaming in and out of the fitness center? One of the difference-makers in their journey toward health is if they are traveling *with friends*. Those with a small group of companions at their side are much more likely to stay in it for the long haul and have fun at the same time. That is the power of community. You and your Growth Group will move from fitness to wellness, from nutrition to wholeness, and from health all the way to life!

The holistic approach to *Living Wellness for Growth Groups* reminds me of something . . . Jesus was once asked, "What is the greatest commandment?" Quoting words from the Old Testament, he answered, "Love the Lord your God with all your heart and with all your soul and with all your strength and with all your mind" (Luke 10:27). To love God might easily be considered just a soul issue, or maybe a heart issue. But Jesus also saw it as something to be done with all your strength and with all your mind. He blew the regular categories out of the water and saw you and me as *whole people* created in the image of God. What if we applied the same lesson to fitness and nutrition?

What if we invited the spirit and the mind into this conversation about the body? Well, this is it!

As profound as *Living Wellness for Growth Groups* will be for you, it is remarkably straightforward and easy to grasp. In these pages, you will find out why you need certain nutrients to be fit and healthy and why others harm your body. You will see illustrated step-by-step workouts and stretching pages, and you will read about the honest need we all have for spiritual health. You will be inspired to change what needs changing in your life, and you will have some trusted friends on the road with you to cheer you on!

You have discovered a gem. Read it, live it, and share it with others. Be blessed!

—BJORN DIXON, MDiv, pastor of the WHY Church in Elk River, Minnesota

INTRODUCTION

Dear Friend,

As I write this, I'm listening to a cricket chirp in my basement. He has been there for some time now—days, maybe even a week. He chirps on and off all day. I imagine how he longs to be set free. There are no other crickets down there with him. He cries out in vain. I have tried rescuing this cricket a few times. I heard him chirping as I descended the stairs and I thought, *This is going to be easy*. However, as soon as I stepped onto the floor, the chirping stopped. I waited a minute to see if he would give his position away. No, he would not. Back up the stairs for me. Ten minutes later, the lonely chirping began again. Once more, I headed down the stairs, more quietly this time. The same thing happened, although I was able to get closer before he went silent. I wanted to set the cricket free, but his fear was holding him captive. As I write this letter to you, the lonely cricket serenades me (or if I'm honest with myself, irritates me).

I wonder how often you and I are like this cricket. When we finally take the time to self-reflect, we find ourselves in a place we didn't imagine or want to be, perhaps thirty pounds overweight after a first child or struggling with the same ten pounds over and over again; wrestling with depression, anxiety, or self-worth; or stuck in a meaningless job because we don't have the courage or strength to start over. Friends, if you are examining your life and health and you find yourself chirping in a basement, take heart! You are not alone! You have a heavenly father who is waiting for you to sit down and learn from him—and then take action.

Living Wellness for Growth Groups includes scripture and reflection for your spiritual growth. Whether you are new to the idea of faith and don't really know who Jesus is, or you have attended church your whole life and have a deep faith in Christ—wherever you are in your faith walk, trust that God longs to draw you deeper into a relationship with him. He longs to heal your mind, body, and spirit and set you free from whatever holds you back from an abundant life (2 Corinthians 3:17, John 8:36, John 10:10).

Freedom, balance, and abundant life are just a few joys I find in Jesus. I have discovered and am excited to share the good news that my journey to faith includes all elements of my health, including physical fitness and nutritional choices. *Living Wellness for Growth Groups* is based on my own health experiences, the experiences of thousands of successful clients, and years of research from leading experts in the field (quoted throughout the book). The program focuses on three main elements:

1. Nutrition (the art of eating for nourishment, rather than for fuel alone)

2. Fitness (I call it "happy movement" because I encourage you to find something enjoyable)

3. Faith (encouragement and support from the Creator of your body!)

If you're taking this journey with a small group, I encourage you to be authentic with them. Proverbs 15:22 says, "Plans fail for lack of counsel, but with many advisers they succeed." Dialogue with other participants is one key to success with this program. We were not meant to travel this path alone.

If you're taking this journey independently (not in a small group), I encourage you to find a trusted friend or mentor. Ask him or her if you can work through the reflection questions together.

You are beginning one of the most important journeys of your life. *Living Wellness for Growth Groups* is a book that looks at the health of your mind, body, spirit, and heart. Your health affects every part of your life: your finances (and your ability to give), your relationships with others (and your ability to serve), your economic footprint (and the earth you will leave for the next generation), and your relationship with God (your intimacy with him depends on spending time in his presence) in all areas of your life, *including your physical health*. Your path will be full of small hills and what may feel like giant mountains. But every step will bring you closer to who you were created to be if you daily invite God into your journey and respond to his prompting.

Take your time. Go through the book a little each day or set aside a larger chunk of time and tackle the whole week at once. Either way is fine (although I think reading and writing a little each day is most effective).

But don't just *read* the questions in this book; *write out* your responses to each one. I have gone through book studies before, reading and thinking, *That's a great question*. But when I actually stopped and wrote out my answers, the results were *life-changing*.

My mission is to *revolutionize health, one community at a time*. This is a big goal, and you are a critical part of my mission. My soul grieves when I see people suffering from preventable illness, disease, and cancer. How much greater will our relationships be with improved health? Who will we become without the shame of unrealistic body image and pretending to be who we're not?

You can do this! You can change. As Bill Hybels says, "You've got to have grit to be a leader." You are the leader of your health and well-being. You are the only person who can make you healthier. Being healthier is challenging, and it's not for the faint of heart. You're going to struggle and make mistakes. You're going to take two steps forward and one step back. *But there is grace, so much grace*. This journey is more about who you're *becoming* than what you're *doing*. God has important plans for your life, and God is "able to do immeasurably more than all we ask or imagine, according to his power that is at work within us, to him be glory in the church and in Christ Jesus throughout all generations, for ever and ever! Amen." (Ephesians 3:20–21)

Instead of becoming silent when you hear footsteps on the stairs, keep chirping! God is waiting for you, *within* reach. This is your chance to make lasting changes in your health and well-being. This journey is about living. This journey is about wellness. Why?

You are worth more than mediocre. You are worth *exceptional* health.

Praying for you,

Ashley R. Darkenwald

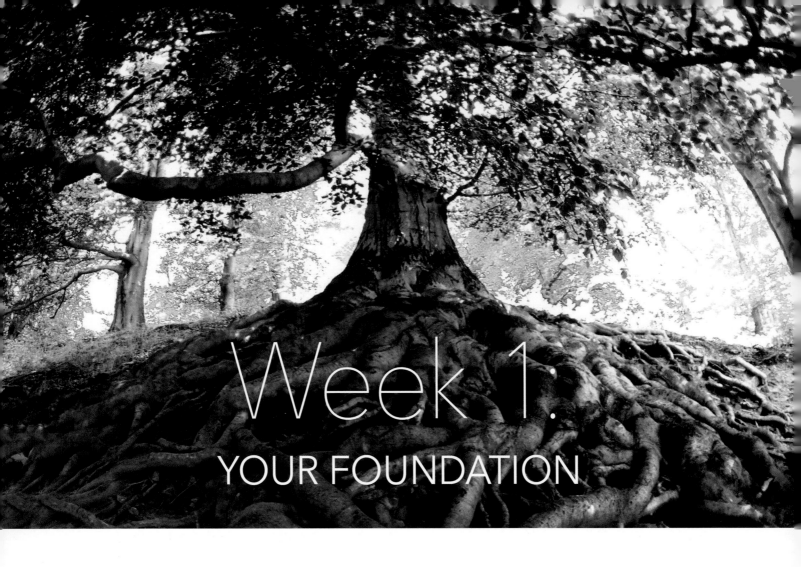

Week 1:
YOUR FOUNDATION

To conclude the sermon on the mount, where Jesus gives instructions on how to live an abundant life, he tells a parable about two people: one who built a house on sand and one who built a house on rock. When turbulent weather came, the house with the firm foundation was the only one left standing.

Your foundation, physically, emotionally, and spiritually, determines your ability to weather life when it gets rough.

This week, we are laying a strong foundation that will allow us to live abundantly, despite our circumstances.

Just because something has always been does not mean it will always be.

Week1, Day 1: Getting Started!

Welcome to *Living Wellness for Growth Groups*! Congratulate yourself for investing in your health. We will spend the next eight weeks together learning about the inner workings of our body and the connectedness of our body, mind, spirit, *and God.* And of course, we will be practicing what we learn.

What Are Living Wellness Growth Groups?

Living Wellness Growth Groups are a new approach to achieving a *healthy balance* of one's mind, body, and spirit. Rather than just focusing on weight loss, growth group participants find lasting health through discovering their 'root why.' Think about a tree with deep roots underground. When we begin to answer self-examining questions, we often think of the first thing that pops into our minds. These are often surface answers. When we dig a little deeper, under the surface, we begin to find our roots, our motives behind our decisions. Your ideals about health started when you were very young. Why do you make the choices you do? What causes lasting change? Who is God calling you to be in this season? Together, we will examine these questions *and more* over the next eight weeks.

Living Wellness Growth Groups provide a safe space for people *to be* and *become* who God created them to be. The growth groups are similar to small-group book studies, where participants come to discuss and discover what happens when one connects the health of his or her whole body, mind, and spirit. But the group doesn't end with discussion. The format includes a grocery store tour, hands-on practice, journaling, stretching and exercise, and daily accountability.

No matter where you are in your journey, your health plays a major role in your ability to fulfill God's purpose for your life. Achieving balance in our lives becomes clear when our desires fade away as God's desires for our lives take the driver's seat.

Living Wellness Growth Groups create space for self-reflection and discovery that will take you *from fitness to wellness, from nutrition to wholeness, and from health all the way to abundant life!* Every step of this journey will bring you closer to who you are created to be if you daily invite God into your struggles and accomplishments. We are inviting God into our health journey and asking another question, *"What does it look like for me to live an abundant life"?* This revelation is what we desire to explore with you!

Living Wellness Five Keys to Success

Living Wellness Growth Group participants have discovered sustainable health through the five keys of success. These keys set Living Wellness apart by creating a community environment focused on growth for your long-term success.

Knowledge—The foundational knowledge in this book will help guide your health and wellness choices. There is no one-size-fits-all approach. When you know how your inner body works and which foods nourish or harm you, you will be able to make informed and empowered decisions.

Mindfulness—We create new, healthy habits once we recognize and throw away old, destructive habits. We will practice mindfulness in all areas of our lives, from how we eat and exercise to how we think about ourselves and our bodies. Mindfulness creates awareness. Awareness opens up doors.

Accountability—We are not alone in this journey. We are held accountable to ourselves, one another, and God. We will lift one another up when we fall and encourage one another when we succeed. Accountability keeps us on the path when we don't feel like moving forward.

Inspiration—A small drop of water can be seen through its ripple on the other side of the ocean! Living Wellness Growth Group participants consistently become inspired when they acquire the knowledge, become accountable to one another, become more mindful about their decisions, and understand their motivations for their actions. Living Wellness Growth Groups have been designed to inspire you for lasting change by igniting intentions into action, and empowering you to step into the person God created you to be. We trust you will be inspired too.

Motivation—Through practice, discussion, and reflection, we discover the big "why" behind what we do. The root "why" is simply asking the question "why" multiple times until we find the source of our motivations. When we know our true motives for doing something, rather than our surface answers or excuses, we are more likely to achieve success with our health goals *long term*.

SMART Goals

Each week, you will state your health and wellness intentions by writing out your action steps (goals) in this book. Set yourself up for success by using specific, measurable, achievable, relevant, and time-bound goals. Use the following principles when setting your weekly strength, cardio, and nutrition action steps.

Specific—I often hear participants set weekly goals to "eat healthier" or "get stronger." These seem like good goals for a health and wellness group, but how tangible are they? How do you measure if you ate healthier or got stronger? In order to identify a successful attempt at a goal, your goals need to be as *specific* as possible. Rather than writing to "eat healthier," you may make a goal to eat *two different colored vegetables each day for the next week*. That's a specific goal—and it certainly will result in eating healthier!

Measureable—If one of your goals is to "drink more water" and I ask you the following week if you drank more water, you may respond, "I think so." In order to track your progress and know what strategies work for you, you must make *measurable* goals. If your goal is to drink more water each day, set a measureable amount—say, *twenty more ounces of water per day* or so. With a measureable goal, you'll be able analyze if you achieved your goal, and if you did not, you can make a new plan of attack.

Achievable—Be realistic. Living Wellness Growth Groups are not reality TV shows where you exercise seven hours per day and live on carrots. Participants who see the greatest short- and long-term results set small, attainable goals. The more achievable your goals, the more courage you will have to set new goals and accomplish them! In the measureable section I stated an example goal of drinking twenty more ounces of water per day. Ultimately, your goal is to drink half of your ideal body weight in ounces of filtered water every day. But, if that's new to you, it would be wise to start with a more achievable goal, such as an additional twenty ounces of water per day. Give yourself grace. Be your own best friend. You are worth it!

Relevant—Be sure your goals relate to the health and wellness of your mind, body, and spirit. Review your goals periodically to ensure they are still relevant. For example, once you are consistently drinking more water, increase your goal. Each week as you set new action steps, review your previous weeks' action steps. Adjust your upcoming goals accordingly.

Time-bound—When will you accomplish your goal? Is this a one-week or an eight-week goal? Set a time frame around your goal so that it doesn't become a bucket-list item when it should just be a short-term venture.

Stages of Change

For every change you go through in life, you travel through stages of change. You may go through some stages in thirty seconds or less while some may take years; for most people, this is a subconscious process. They don't recognize the process of moving between the stages. But in order to make realistic goals, you must identify what stage you are currently in for each particular goal. These stages are adapted from James Prochaska, professor of psychology and director of the Cancer Prevention Research Center at the University of Rhode Island and developer of the Transtheoretical Model of Behavior Change beginning in 1977.

Pre-contemplation (sometimes known as denial)—In this stage, you are not ready for change. You usually blame others for your health obstacles or problems. You may make such statements as, "I couldn't work out this week because it was raining," or, "I couldn't eat well because I was at my in-laws' house." You haven't (or don't want to) come to grips with your current situation, and this keeps you from moving into the next stage of change. Can you think of an area in your health where you are in denial? Sometimes it helps to ask a trusted friend—denial is easier to point out in someone else than in ourselves!

Contemplation—You are now thinking about changing. This requires hope! You must *believe* you can change in order to create a foundation for lasting change. In this stage, you start thinking about what your life will look like with a new habit or behavior. You think about taking the next steps and making the change happen. What are you contemplating changing with your health?

Preparation—This is where you prepare to take action. You buy the water bottle, get the gym membership, plan a new routine, make a grocery list, or set aside time for meal planning. This is an exciting stage, but be aware! You could stay in pre-contemplation, contemplation, and preparation your whole life (let's not!). If you're not currently exercising, it may be a good idea to spend some time *preparing* to exercise. For example, your cardio action step for next week may be to *plan out* an exercise routine *and* a backup plan if your first attempt goes sideways. Use this stage to discover what works well for you and what does not.

Action—*This is easier than you think!* Take a leap of faith and trust that God will give you the strength to *take action*. You can do this! This is the stage where you *drink* the water, *work out* at the gym (or at home), *stick* to a routine, and/or *grocery shop* for healthy foods. Setting small, achievable goals and returning to them no matter how many times you fall off the wagon leads to long-term success. Consistent action creates habits, or maintenance.

Maintenance—Our actions become routine, habit. You don't have to think about brushing your teeth anymore (hopefully!), because you have created a habit. Let's get to maintenance with every one of our health goals *one goal at a time!* Slow and steady wins the health race.

Relapse—The most significant stage of change because what you do with your relapse or set back determines the longevity of your success. *Everyone* relapses in some area of his or her life at some point. Just because you relapse *does not mean you are starting over*! Take heart! Usually, you just need to be mindful of your current circumstance and think, *what changed*? Did your normal routine change? Did the weather change? Did you get ill or injured? This is life. Take a breath. Call a friend. And make a new plan. *You are worth the time it takes to get back on that wagon and move forward with your health!*

Brainstorm your top health and wellness goals. Some examples may be to have less pain, to get better sleep, to eat more vegetables, to lose weight, to start exercising, and so on. Write them here.

To ~~loose~~ lose weight, feel better, more energy, sleep better, handle stress better, get healthy, start a family, improve my marriage, decrease pain, be more active, enjoy life.

Circle one. What stage of change are you in with that particular goal? Please explain why you feel you are in that stage.

I am really ready to make a change - I'm Preparation/Action plan. I am trying new methods to become healthier by reading books/mags, online sites/groups, internet searches and more!

Intro to Managing Your Weight

One small but important aspect of being a healthy person is to have an understanding of calories—the basic unit of energy measured in foods and beverages. The reason you need to have an understanding of calories is because attaining and maintaining a healthy weight is dependent on balancing your caloric input with your output of energy. Consuming more calories than you use will lead to weight gain, obesity, and chronic diseases. On the other hand, consuming too few calories puts the body into starvation mode, which damages the metabolism, slowing down the rate at which your body burns fat as fuel.

I have had clients ask me if they can just consume 500 calories per day to lose two or more pounds per week in order to avoid exercise. The answer is no. This severe calorie deficit is not healthy, and consequently, there is no way to get enough nourishment. See a nutritionist or doctor if you want an exact number to consume (which varies slightly every day).

How can you keep track and balance your calories? Journal!

Keep a Wellness Journal

I have one *strong* recommendation, and it is to keep a detailed wellness journal and count your calories, even for a short period of time. Participants who journal are more successful. Period.

While some programs suggest that no calorie counting is needed to lose weight, those plans are usually so strict that most people cannot adhere to them long term. And because most people have a limited understanding of calories, they end up failing the program. You will learn crucial information about yourself and your eating and exercise habits. You will be held accountable for everything you put in your mouth and all the hours of exercise you do (or don't do!). Even if you have kept a journal in the past, please try again. You are a different person now. *Living Wellness Journals* are available at www.AshleyDarkenwald.com.

If you don't like paper journals, try a fitness application (app) on your smartphone or a calorie- and exercise-tracking website. Finding one that's right for you will help you stick with it.

Counting calories in a journal is one tool to practice on your health journey, not the health journey itself. Calories are the very unit of energy for *all* foods and beverages. We do not need to (and we should not) obsess over calories to have a solid understanding of how many we need and how many calories are in our foods and beverages.

> The ultimate goal of eating is to nourish our bodies.

The ultimate goal of eating is to nourish our bodies. My personal goal is to eat for nourishment 95 percent of the time and reserve that last 5 percent for healthy, natural treats.

The Science Behind Managing Your Weight: Balancing Calories & Nourishment

Use the following formula to calculate how many calories you need to maintain your body weight or how many calories you need to decrease your body fat (weight). The key to balancing a healthy lifestyle without starving or spending clueless hours at the gym is knowing how to eat and exercise to nourish, rather than simply fuel your body. Read on.

Calculating Your Success

1. Calculate your basal metabolic rate (BMR). Your BMR is the amount of energy your body burns doing basic functions, such as breathing and circulating blood. Do the equation in the appropriate formula from left to right. See the section below for examples.

Men *under* age thirty, do this equation:

(0.0621 × your weight) ÷ 2.2 + 2.0357 = _____ × 240 = _____ × 1.05 = _____ BMR

Women *under* age thirty, do this equation:

(0.0621 × your weight) ÷ 2.2 + 2.0357 = _____ × 240 = _____ BMR

Men *over* age thirty, do this equation:

(0.0342 × your weight) ÷ 2.2 + 3.5377 = _____ × 240 = _____ × 1.05 = _____ BMR

Women *over* age thirty, do this equation:

(0.0342 × your weight) ÷ 2.2 + 3.5377 = _7.28_ × 240 = _1748_ BMR

1. What is your <u>average</u> daily activity level? Circle one. **Do not count exercise:**

    a. Sedentary (i.e., driving or desk job): Factor: 1.1
    b. Lightly active (i.e., nurse or teacher): Factor: 1.2 *(circled)*
    c. Heavily active (i.e., server or construction): Factor: 1.3

2. Multiply your BMR and your activity level (use the appropriate factor based off your activity level: 1.1, 1.2, *or* 1.3). This is your approximate number of calories to maintain your current body weight:

    _1748_ BMR × _1.2_ Activity Factor = _2097_ Your Maintenance Calories

Female Example

Let's look at an example of a BMR equation for a forty-five-year-old female who weighs 180 pounds.

1. (0.0342 x 180) ÷ 2.2 + 3.5377 = 6.34 × 240 = 1,521.6

2. Sedentary lifestyle = 1.1 factor

3. 1,520 (rounded) × 1.1 = 1,672 is the approximate number our female example needs to maintain her current weight (maintenance calories).

Male Example

Let's look at an example of a BMR equation for a forty-five-year-old male who weighs 200 pounds.

1. $(0.0342 \times \underline{200}) \div 2.2 + 3.5377 = \underline{6.65} \times 240 \times 1.05 = \underline{1,675.8}$
2. Lightly active = 1.2 factor
3. 1,675 (rounded) × 1.2 = 2,010 is the approximate number our male example needs to maintain his current weight (maintenance calories).

Maintenance calories indicate that if you eat that amount of calories per day without exercising, you will not gain or lose weight. You will maintain your current body weight.

How Do You Decrease Body Fat?

To decrease body fat, you need a calorie deficit. You must consume fewer than your maintenance calories and/or burn more calories than you consume with daily activity and exercise. Each of our bodies are unique. There are multiple factors that contribute to our nutritional needs.

Recent research is demonstrating that the rate at which one will lose weight is slower than previously thought. Studies are also finding that it's common to plateau after a certain period of weight loss. The factors contributing to these occurrences are complicated, but they include noncompliance to the plan and a lack of recalculating caloric needs once weight loss occurs. You may use an online tool to determine your calorie needs and expected schedule of weight loss.

We encourage you to use the guidelines below, to track your progress and adjust accordingly. Your calorie needs should be reassessed with every ten pounds lost or gained *or* once you hit your target weight.

The section below will help you approximate your caloric needs based on the assumption that a 3,500-calorie surplus or deficit equals one pound of body fat gained or lost, respectively. To use this basic formula for a weight loss goal of one pound per week, divide 3,500 calories by 7 days, which equals a 500-calorie deficit needed per day. *This 500-calorie deficit can be attained by eating less and/or exercising.*

EXAMPLE: If your maintenance calories are 2,010 and your goal is to lose one pound of body fat per week, you could eat 300 less calories, making your calorie goal 1,710. Additionally, you could exercise off 200 calories, creating a total caloric deficit of 500 per day. See Appendix M for a chart of activities and approximate calories burned.

I know you hear stories of people losing five or more pounds per week, but unless they're doing hours and hours *and hours* of exercise *each day* and severely limiting their calories, they're likely experiencing loss of water weight, food, and muscle *in addition* to body fat. Look at the chart below to get a better understanding of pounds lost *or gained* as they relate to calories.

Calories—Let's Manage Expectations

The following chart breaks down weight loss by desired number of pounds per week and how many calories you need to reduce per day and week. Between exercise and eating less, the chart offers examples of how combinations of calorie deficits can lead to weight loss.

Remember 3,500 calories = approximately 1 pound of body fat lost or gained.

I don't recommend a daily calorie deficit from nutrition of more than 500 to 800 calories. It is generally accepted that women should not consume fewer than approximately 1,200 to 1,500 calories per day, and men should not consume fewer than approximately 1,500 to 1,800 calories per day. Remember you need fuel *and* nourishment, and if you consume too few calories, you are not nourishing your body. Instead, incorporate more exercise into your daily routine. If your goal is weight loss, write down the number of pounds you want to lose per week.

After equating in the chart below, if your daily calorie intake is less than the recommended, adjust your chart to include more of a deficit from exercise.

Pounds of Body Fat Lost Per Week	Approximate Calorie Deficit Needed Per Day	Daily Exercise Deficit	Daily Calorie Deficit from Nutrition	Total Calorie Deficit Per Week
½	250	125	125	1,750
1	500	250	250	3,500
2	1,000	500	500	7,000
3 (not recommended)	1,500	1,000	500	10,500
Personal Application				

The encouragement for weight loss is in the long game! Any calorie deficit will result in weight loss, but to sustain it, find a calorie balance that leaves you *feeling satisfied*, realistically managing your expectations, and getting back up if you stumble.

Weight Loss Calorie Goal

To determine your daily calorie intake, calculate the following:

_____ (maintenance calories) - _____ (calorie deficit from nutrition) =

_____ (daily calorie intake)

If you do *not* desire to lose weight, this number should be the same as your maintenance calorie number.

Again, it is my strongest recommendation that you spend these next eight weeks learning and journaling about how much energy (calories) is in the foods you eat and drink.

Once you recognize your body's needs, you will no longer need to keep track of calories, water, exercise, and how you feel on a regular basis! One of the most important (and satisfying) health goals is to learn your body's needs so you can respond when your body speaks to you. Intuitive health is the ability to *listen and respond* to the signals, symptoms, and needs of your body.

> Intuitive health is the ability to listen and respond to the signals, symptoms, and needs of your body.

Time to Get Fit!

Cardiovascular training, strength training, and stretching are three fitness components we'll be focusing on over the next eight weeks. Our goal is not to get you running marathons by the end of week eight. It's for you to do more physical activity and to create a routine that you enjoy. We will be looking at each of these components in more detail below.

Light Physical Activity –
Start here if you're not currently exercising

You should move your body every day. This is no news flash, but even though the benefits are so immense, we still choose to sit more than move. Light physical activity keeps our joints lubricated, increases circulation, and prevents arthritis; these benefits are an active recipe for physical longevity.

Start moving every day to create healthy habits. Examples of physical activity include:

- Walking—Take a family walk or walk your dog before dinner every night (walking alone is great too!).
- Dancing—Do this after dinner while cleaning the kitchen. Turn on your favorite music and move while you work!
- Playing recreational sports—Look for adult recreation teams in your community: volleyball, softball, golf, and the like. These adult sports are a great way to get active and meet people in your community with similar interests!
- Raking leaves—Make leaf houses with the neighbor kids.
- House cleaning—Need I say more? Don't forget the music!

Many of these activities can be turned into cardio training when you get your heart rate up to at least 65 percent of your maximum heart rate.

Cardio Training

Did you know your body contains 50,000 to 100,000 miles of arteries and veins?! Given that your cardiovascular system is so vast, you must take care of your heart in order to make it last.

The benefits of cardio training include:

- Strengthening your heart muscle and blood vessels
- Preventing issues like heart disease, high blood pressure, and diabetes
- Strengthening the immune system
- Achieving and maintaining a healthy body weight
- Increasing metabolism
- Releasing "feel good" hormones
- Increasing the rate at which your body heals itself
- Reducing muscle soreness when performed after strength training

To improve your current fitness level, the National Academy of Sports Medicine recommends adding a *minimum of thirty minutes per day, three to five times per week of cardiovascular exercise.* Several short cardio workouts (ten- to fifteen-minute spurts at different times in one day) can be just as effective as one long cardio workout. Set your goals based on your current physical activity level.

Your goal as a Living Wellness Growth Group participant is to do more cardio exercise than you're currently doing. If you're not currently exercising, adding three to ten minutes of cardio exercise per day would be a great start! You'll be setting goals each week for your cardio training in your action steps.

Below are some examples of activities that can elevate the heart rate into the cardio zone:

• Cycling • Jumping rope • Running (4–6 MPH) • Rowing (fast) • Brisk walking

• Mountain biking • Swimming • Elliptical training • Skiing • Weight lifting (circuit style)

Be sure to check your heart rate during exercise to ensure you are in a cardio zone.

Which of these cardio activities appeal to you?

Calculating Your Heart Rate Zones

How do you calculate your heart rate zones? Below is a simple way to find your maximum heart rate (MHR) and your approximate heart rate zones. Your MHR is the upper limit of what your cardiovascular system can handle for short periods of time during physical activity. Heart rate zones are math equations; they show how to monitor how hard your heart is working. If you're training for a specific race or event, I would recommend using the Karvonen Formula (not shown), which factors in your resting heart rate.

Calculating your heart rate (cardio) zones: What is your age? _____

Max Heart Rate (MHR): 220 -_____ age = _____ MHR

Zone 1 = 65-75% of your MHR: _____ Beats Per Minute (BPM) (Warm up and cool down zone. You should feel in control—you could stay in this zone for more than two hours.)

Zone 2 = 76-85% of your MHR: _____ BPM (You should feel challenged—**the majority of your cardio workout should be in this zone**—you could safely work out here for twenty minutes to two hours.)

Zone 3 = 86-95% MHR: _____ BPM (You should feel as though you want out—you should not stay in this for more than two minutes.)

Remember, it's important to have an understanding of your heart rate zones so you know if you're working hard enough to meet your goals or if you're working too hard and stressing your heart.

Let's practice taking your pulse. Pull up the stopwatch feature on your phone or look at a clock with a second hand. Take your pulse for six seconds. Add a zero to that number to get your estimated BPM. For example, if you counted seven beats in six seconds, your heart rate would be 70 BPM. For a more accurate number, count your pulse for thirty seconds and double that number to get your BPM.

Write your resting heart rate here: _____ BPM. Be sure to calculate your BPM occasionally during different points in your exercise to determine what zone you're in. Adjust your workout accordingly.

Strength Training

Another key aspect of fitness is strength training. The benefits of strength training include improving:

- Overall muscular strength
- Core strength
- Bone mineral density
- Muscular endurance
- Joint stability and range of motion
- Control of your posture
- Body image
- Neuromuscular efficiency (balance and stabilization together)

To improve your strength, add a minimum of twenty minutes two to three times per week of strength training.

Living Wellness Growth Group participants, you'll receive videos demonstrating exercises over the next eight weeks.

Additionally, there are four full body strength training workouts in Appendix L. Use these proven and effective workouts, based off the National Academy of Sports Medicine Optimum Performance Training (OPT) training model guidelines to change up your current strength routine. Muscles adapt to the same workout after four to six weeks, but feel free to change it up every two weeks to avoid boredom.

If this sounds overwhelming, a great place to start is to simply do the two exercises in week 1 as your strength routine. Each week's material provides additional exercises. Add them to your routine to eventually create a full body workout.

Two Birds, One Dumbbell: Cardio and Strength Together

Cardio and strength training can be accomplished simultaneously. Circuit training is performing one strength exercise after another with minimal rest (twenty seconds or less) in between exercises. This type of training elevates the heart rate to zone two for the duration of the workout. Remember, for cardio benefits, you should aim to do this style of workout for a minimum of ten minutes at a time.

Stretching and Foam Rolling

Stretching is *as important* as cardio and strength training. Please do not neglect this important aspect of your health for time's sake. I would rather have you shorten your workout in order to include stretching than skip it to get more of a cardio or strength workout.

Stretching can be accomplished through light, static holding of the muscle in a lengthened position and through self-myofascial release (foam rolling). Foam rolling is a stretching technique that applies pressure from a cylinder shaped foam to a knot in the muscle.

Please allow time for stretching and foam rolling! Stretching is vital for:

- Improved flexibility
- Increased energy
- Injury prevention
- Muscle, joint, and bone health
- Eliminating tight muscles prior to workout
- Full range of motion
- Maximal strength gains
- Increased relaxation

Research from the National Academy of Sports Medicine suggests that you can stretch tight muscles before you work out. After you work out, stretch the muscles you just worked. I recommend stretching your muscles every day. Another great time to stretch is when you need to take a break from sitting and/or doing repetitive movements.

Refer to Appendix L for a full range of foam roll and stretching exercises. Hold each stretch for at least thirty seconds or five to seven deep breaths.

Week 1 Action Steps & Check-in Partner Guidelines

Each week, you will fill out action steps. These are your objectives for the week. You will fill out the top three with your check-in partner and the rest individually. Check-in partners should be male-male and female-female only (unless you're a couple going through this together and you *want* to be partners). You are encouraged to exchange contact information with your partner and check in with him or her *daily*. This person will be your check-in partner for the week. Each week, connect with a new check-in partner if possible.

If male-male and female-female check-in partners are not possible within your group or you're going through this study on your own, seek out a trusted friend or mentor who is ahead of you in his or her health journey and ask that person to check in with you daily.

Below are a few thoughts as you embark on this accountability journey.

1. Be honest with your check-in partner.
2. Be gracious; remember no one is perfect.
3. Be willing to ask for help with a goal that's more challenging than anticipated.
4. Be encouraging and inspiring to one another.

1. Check in with your partner daily.

    a. Partner's name and contact info: _____

2. Record your **strength** workouts in the *Living Wellness Journal**; weekly goal:

    _____ _____ (number of days) (minutes per day)

    a. Partner's goal: _____ _____ (number of days) (minutes per day)

3. Record your **cardio** workouts in the *Living Wellness Journal*; weekly goal:

    _____ _____

    a. Partner's goal: _____ _____

4. Record your **food/beverage** intake in an app or the *Living Wellness Journal*

5. If you have not already done so, complete the health and wellness survey online at www. AshleyDarkenwald.com.

6. Read and fill out all questions for week 1.**

Living Wellness Journal and other resources are available at www.AshleyDarkenwald.com.

**This week, the reading and questions will take about fifteen to twenty minutes per day to complete. Subsequent weeks will take about half the time to complete. This is your foundation! Give yourself the time you deserve for this journey.

Would you pray with me as we close out this day?

Dear God, thank you for the opportunity to be healthier. Thank you for your unconditional love and grace. Please be with us as we walk through this new health journey. Please give us the wisdom to listen and the strength and courage to step into action where you lead. We trust in your goodness. We love you. Amen.

Week 1, Day 2: Spiritual and Physical Disciplines – Discovering Your Happy Movement (Exercise)

List as many spiritual disciplines that come to mind:

_____

_____

_____

You may have written such things as prayer, reading scripture, going to church, fasting, and the like.

Are any of these things required to come into a right relationship with Jesus Christ?

No. God says we are saved by grace alone—not by what we do but by what Jesus did on the cross for us. In addition to having been saved by grace, we have a beautiful opportunity to live in obedience to God in all areas of our lives. Asking God into your health journey (mind, body, and spirit) is the first step to being obedient to God with your health. The next step is to listen to where he's leading you and then take action! Ultimately, this leads to abundant life.

It is out of our lavish love for God that we devote our lives to him and discipline ourselves in order to trust God, grow in our faith, and bear fruit.

This is also true of our physical disciplines. Must we exercise to survive? No. Will we die if we don't strengthen our muscles? No.

In 1 Corinthians 9:27, the apostle Paul says, "I discipline my body like an athlete, training it to do what it should. Otherwise, I fear that after preaching to others I myself might be disqualified."

Why would Paul give this encouragement, and why do so many of us take our physical health for granted? Just as prayer is a discipline that brings us closer to God, so is taking care of our physical bodies. We bear the image of God. How we take care of our physical bodies looks different to each person, but we can all do our part to care for the bodies we've been given.

Do you think your physical health is important for vibrant spiritual health? Why?

_____

_____

_____

God sees how we handle all the details of our lives. Luke 16:10 states: "If you are faithful in little things, you will be faithful in large ones. But if you are dishonest in little things, you won't be honest with greater responsibilities." Let's be excellent stewards of our physical health. With this revelation in mind, let's look at a few guidelines on how to best care for our physical health.

The minimum guidelines for physical exercise are as follows:

According to the American Heart Association, heart attack and stroke are the number-one and number-five killers in America. Below are the 2015 guidelines for the minimum exercise recommendation.

For Overall Cardiovascular Health:

- At least **30 minutes of moderate-intensity** aerobic activity at least **5 days per week for a total of 150 minutes**

OR

- At least **25 minutes of vigorous** aerobic activity at least **3 days per week for a total of 75 minutes**; or a combination of moderate- and vigorous-intensity aerobic activity

AND

- **Moderate- to high-intensity muscle-strengthening activity** at least **2 days per week** for additional health benefits.

For Lowering Blood Pressure and Cholesterol

- An average of **40 minutes of moderate- to vigorous-intensity** aerobic activity **3 or 4 times per week**

These guidelines are not in place to make us miserable—quite the opposite, actually. Following these guidelines can keep our hearts healthy, our lungs and arteries strong, our bones and joints mobile, and our energy levels high.

People tell me all the time that they don't have the energy or motivation to work out, when in reality, the workout is what clears the brain and gives people energy! Regular exercise also reduces stress, lowers blood pressure, manages weight, and releases endorphins (natural feel-good chemicals in the brain).

If you're currently inactive, start small.

I have not always been fit and healthy. In high school, I decided to change course from a three-season athlete to a theater performer. This dramatically reduced my activity level, and I gained weight. If you had asked my friends, they would not have classified me as overweight, but you can imagine the surprise when I lost twenty pounds in college from a consistent running routine! I did not start out running miles and miles per day. I made a commitment to get to the gym every day for at least **three minutes**. Yes, just three minutes. I heard a motivational speaker say that anyone can make time for three minutes per day for something important. I was working full time to pay for college and taking a substantial course load to graduate early.

Three minutes per day of exercise for one semester: This simple commitment developed into a habit and a discipline for physical fitness that led to my unforeseen weight loss, rejuvenated interest in health, and passion for helping others find their start to a lifelong journey of health and whole-person wellness. Back then, running was my happy movement. Today, my happy movement is biking, kayaking, lifting weights, and playing recreational volleyball. It's ok if your happy movement is different today than it used to be.

The big question is—what should *you* do for *your* happy movement?

The big answer is—*whatever exercise you'll do!* Find your *happy movement*, something you enjoy (or at least tolerate), and do it. Nike hit it right on the head with their slogan: Just Do It.

Swim
Bike
Walk
Golf
Run
Dance
Lift
Stretch
Play a sport
Mix it up!
Just move

The key to creating lifelong healthy habits is to move your body *every day*. Make your movements challenging, but achievable. If you have the resources, spend some time with a fitness professional to learn how to work out properly and how to stretch your muscles. The exercises in this book help you understand proper form and get a full body workout. Use the instructions given to exercise safely.

Tips to Get Started:

1. Start right now. Do not wait one more minute. Pick something you enjoy and can do safely (walk) and do it right now. Are you injured? In a wheelchair? You can still sit and strengthen your upper body.

2. Get support. Find a walking buddy, swimming pal, or fellow lifter. Encourage your check-in partner during these eight weeks together and ask for accountability with your happy movement in return. Get strong together. Get your kids involved with

your physical fitness, or get active while they're in activities. Walk laps at the baseball practice or hit the gym while they have dance. Avoid using other people's schedules as an excuse for you to be inactive.

3. Invite God into your physical health journey.

Pray with me:

Dear God, thank you for the gift of my body. Please give me the desire to honor you with my physical health. Forgive me for not taking care of my physical body in the past. Please show me how you desire me to honor you with my choices and my time.

Living Wellness Videos

1. For those just getting started in strength training, this is a great way to get started.
2. For those currently strength training, you'll gain new ideas.
3. Learn correct form—three push-ups in good form are better than ten push-ups in bad form.

Living Wellness Week 1 Exercises

Over the course of the next eight weeks, you will be practicing pieces of one full strength training workout. This workout is found in its entirety in Appendix L.

Lunge to Balance

Inhale as you step forward or backward into your lunge—tightening the glute on your rear leg. Exhale as you step up into a balance posture. Hold your balance for at least two seconds, pulling your belly button into your spine, and squeezing your gluteal muscles (butt) as you keep your core tight.

For Option II, add a biceps curl as you lift your leg into the balance position.

Perform 16 to 20 lunges on each leg. Repeat as time permits. Practice every other day.

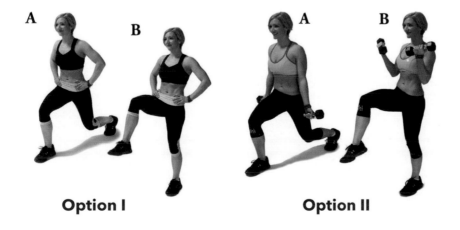

Option I   **Option II**

Push-Ups

From the tabletop posture (hands and knees), make sure your wrists are directly beneath your shoulders, your back is straight, your abdominals are sucked in, and your glutes are tight. Inhale as you bend your arms, keeping your core straight and tight, and exhale as you push your arms straight, rounding out your upper back at the top of the push-up. Do not allow your back to arch. If push-ups hurt your back, stop immediately. If you have no pain in a different position, practice them against a wall or table.

For Option II, perform your push-ups from your toes.

Perform 16 to 20 push-ups. Repeat as time permits. Practice every other day. Remember to stretch after your workout.

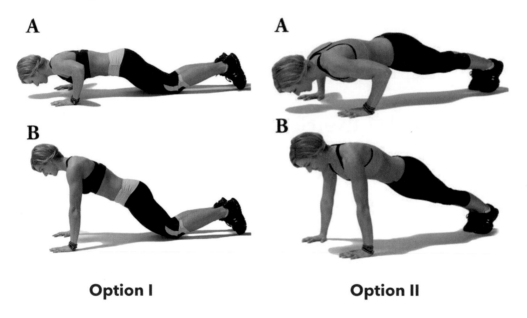

Option I   **Option II**

How might you live a more abundant life if you honored God with your physical health?

_____

_____

_____

What happy movement will you commit to this week to practice physical discipline?

_____

_____

_____

_____

Week 1, Day 3: Trusting God's Best for Your Health

I trust God when he says he wants the best for me and my life (Jeremiah 29:11). I trust God when he says he wants me to have a full, abundant life (John 10:10). I didn't always trust him, though. Especially when it came to my health. I trusted myself, my doctors, and my over-the-counter medications to keep me functioning, because, let's face it, that's what I saw everyone else doing. Well, it turns out God has thoughts about being transformed, starting with the renewing of my mind. Read Romans 12:2: "Do not conform to the pattern of this world, but be transformed by the renewing of your mind. Then you will be able to test and approve what God's will is—his good, pleasing and perfect will." When I began trusting God with my health, I had to ask for a new mind-set. I started to think about food and exercise differently. The past several years have been an intentional journey to honor God with my whole life, not just my spiritual life. My health has changed radically since I decided to trust God's best for my life.

In addition to conforming to the traditional American approach to health, do you know what else I used to do? Sabotage my health, suffer unnecessarily, and then pray for healing and restoration. I once described this pattern to someone in a metaphor of banging my head against the wall, repeatedly, then wondering why I had a headache, and then praying for God to cure my headache. When he wouldn't take the pain away, I would take medication. This is called self-sabotage.

Practically, self-sabotage looks like this: I would eat way too much pizza at a social gathering, get a major gut ache the next day, ask God to take the gut ache away, and then take medication for my heartburn. Self-sabotage. The pain was completely preventable! Have you ever been stuck in this cycle?

Your Body Is Designed for Balance

One of the challenges I confront in this industry is individuals who don't feel the need to change their habits because they don't feel terrible or have a chronic disease. When you don't feel terrible, where's the motivation to change? The answer is simple. You don't know what you don't know.

Your body is constantly trying to bring you into a state of homeostasis, or balance. When you eat too much sugar, your body attempts to balance out your blood sugar by releasing insulin into the blood. When you drink soda, your body pulls minerals out of your bones to balance out and bind with the phosphoric acid in the soda. When you don't manage chronic stress, your body releases cortisol to put your body into protection mode, which leads to increased body fat in the midsection. In the short term, these balancing mechanisms are incredibly helpful to keep us functional. But when we don't correct the root of the issue, it's only a matter of time before the body breaks down in a big way.

When we don't know what we don't know, we must trust that God knows what is best for our health. This means having the courage to genuinely ask God to reveal what areas in your life are out of balance and making daily choices that are honoring your body, mind, and spirit.

> When we don't know what we don't know, we must trust that God knows what is best for our health.

Do you trust that your positive fitness and nutrition choices will lead to something more, something better for your health? Circle your answer: Yes / No

I'm not saying that all pain, illness, and diseases can be prevented, but world-renowned scientists (including Preetha Anand et al.) agree in a 2008 *Pharmaceutical Research* article that 90-95 percent of *all* diseases, illnesses, and cancers *are* preventable by our nutrition, fitness, lifestyle choices, and environmental factors, such as smoking, stress, and sleep. Let me repeat, 90-95 percent of *all* diseases, illnesses, and cancers are preventable by our lifestyle and environmental choices!

What would you do for a pill that would take away 95 percent of your physical suffering, never to return again?

The pill is what we put in our mouths, how we move our bodies, and how we manage our stress!

I read a funny coaster in a boutique olive oil store that said: "I'd do anything to lose these ten pounds—except exercise and eat right!" I thought it was funny, at first, because it's so true and generally accepted as normal. But the sad part is, admitting that fact is more acceptable than taking action and being healthier.

Exceptional Health Begins with What You Put into Your Mouth

There's a story in scripture about a rich man who approached Jesus and asked him how to have eternal life. "Jesus answered, 'If you want to be perfect, go, sell your possessions and give to the poor, and you will have treasure in heaven. Then come, follow me'" (Matthew 19:21). The man walked away, sad. The Savior of the world just gave this guy an opportunity of a lifetime—to walk, learn, and eat with the one and only Son of God and, ultimately, have eternal life—and the man walked away.

I wonder what Jesus would say today if he was approached by a person who was tired, overweight, joints aching, and sick all the time. The person might ask, "Jesus, what must I do to have less suffering, a healthy body image, enjoyment of my life, and abundant energy?" Jesus may look at that person with a twinkle in his eye and say, "Honor me with what you put in your mouth. Slow down and eat for nourishment. Rearrange some priorities to become less busy. And honor me with your body by keeping it strong and active. The day will come when I call you into action. You have a purpose and a unique call on your life. Be ready."

Is that person you? How will you reply? Will you trust Jesus and begin the journey to transform your health, make steps to unclutter your life, and make physical exercise a priority?

_____

_____

_____

Friends—God promises to be with you every step of the way (Deuteronomy 31:8).

You can do this. You were created for an abundant, vibrant, fulfilling, healthy life! God promises these things. Do you *trust* him? Take action in the areas of your life and health where you feel him leading you.

Pray with me:

Dearest heavenly father, thank you for your love and this gift of life. Thank you for the gifts of my body, mind, and spirit. Please give me the desire to become the person you created me to be. Forgive me for not trusting you with my health and well-being. Give me the will to be fully yours and fully present on this journey. Amen!

Let's continue your foundational journey by taking an assessment of your health.

Living Wellness Assessment

Your health and wellness story depends on you. Take some time and go through this assessment of your mind, body, and spirit.

Growing up, what was your family's relationship with food, fitness, nutrition, and exercise?

_____

_____

_____

_____

_____

_____

_____

_____

_____

What is your definition of health?

_____

_____

_____

_____

What do you believe can be improved in your health? Examples: your weight, quality or quantity of sleep, amount of vegetables consumed, exercise, and the like.

_____

_____

_____

How will your life change once you improve your physical health? How will you spend your time? Your energy?

_____

_____

_____

What are your top three to five priorities in life?

_____

_____

_____

Being physically unhealthy creates emotional prisons such as low self-confidence and anxiety. In contrast, living an abundant life will help you flourish and be more productive and confident in your job, with your family, and in your social life.

What does an abundant life look like to *you*?

_____

_____

What do you think *God's best* looks like for you in this season of your life?

_____

_____

_____

_____

Your identity plays a role in your ability to live life abundantly. Where does your identity come from?

_____

_____

_____

Nutrition

What are your short-term (one- to eight-week) nutrition goals?

_____

_____

_____

What are your long-term (eight-week to one-year) nutrition goals?

_____

_____

_____

Why is a question we will ask throughout this entire journey. When you ask (and answer) the question "why" authentically, you will discover your motivations or your reasons for doing things. Your motivations for becoming healthier will affect your long-term success. For example, desiring to lose twenty pounds for a reunion may motivate you in the short term, but wanting to be around and active for your grandchildren or not wanting to place preventable burdens on those around you because of failing health will have more of a lasting impact on your long-term health decisions.

Example of asking the root *why*:

Why do you want to be healthy?

> I want to lose twenty pounds.

Why do you want to lose twenty pounds?

> I want to look better.

Why do you want to look better?

> So I feel more confident.

Why do you want to feel more confident?

> So I set a good example for my children.

Why do you want to set a good example for your children?

> So they grow up confident and free to be who God created them to be.

We went from wanting to lose twenty pounds to look better to wanting to lose twenty pounds to set a good example for our children. We still want to lose the twenty pounds, but with the deeper understanding of *why*, we are more likely to achieve and maintain our goals long term.

Why do you want to improve your nutrition?

_____

_____

_____

Why?

_____

_____

_____

Why?

_____

_____

_____

Why?

_____
_____
_____
_____

Why?

_____
_____
_____
_____

What has kept you from achieving your nutrition goals? Be specific.

_____
_____
_____

Weight Loss

We have talked more about weight loss than weight gain as a health goal, because more Americans desire weight loss over weight gain for improved health.

Would losing weight benefit your health? Why?

_____
_____
_____
_____
_____

Please describe everything you ate and drank yesterday with approximate calories (if known). A simple Internet search will help you find your approximate calories:

Food	Calories
Breakfast:	
Snacks:	
Lunch:	
Snacks:	
Dinner:	
Beverages:	
Based on yesterday's account, approximately how many calories are you eating per day?	

Is the above chart a typical day (did you eat more or less than normal)?

_____

_____

_____

_____

Have you tried dieting in the past? If so, how many of the diets yielded lasting results? *Living Wellness for Growth Groups* is *not* a diet. This is a journey of gaining knowledge, accountability, mindfulness, inspiration, and motivation to change your lifestyle.

Remember, there is no one-size-fits-all approach to effective weight management.

Take a look at the food journal you just completed, and your maintenance calorie number from day

1. Are you consuming more calories than you need? Why?

_____

_____

_____

_____

Do you have a history of obsessing over calorie counting or exercise? Which one or both?

_____

_____

_____

Spend time in prayer and ask God to speak to you about your attitude regarding your health and wellness. Ask God for healing in certain areas of your life, if needed.

Nutrition Assessment Continued

How many servings of fruits and veggies did you consume yesterday?

Fruits: _____

Vegetables: _____

Circle if yesterday's total fruit and veggie number is:

less than normal / normal / more than normal

You should consume at least *five to seven servings* of produce each day.

Do you take vitamins or other supplements? Yes/No

List your vitamins or supplements: _____

How much water did you drink yesterday?

_____ Cups or ounces?

Circle: less than normal / normal / more than normal

You should consume half of your ideal body weight in ounces of filtered water every day, plus an additional twenty ounces for every hour you work out.

What is your ideal body weight? _____ Pounds

How much water *should* you be drinking per day? _____ (# lbs. ÷ 2) Ounces

Rate Your Health Activities

Use the chart below to rate each activity. For example, if you practice cardio exercise three times a week for a minimum of thirty minutes, you would put an *X* between *Average* and *Excellent*. This does not have to be exact. Rate how you think you're doing in each category.

Example:	Poor	Average	Excellent
Cardio Exercise		X	
Cardio Exercise			
Strength Exercise			
Vegetable Consumption			
Healthy Fats/Oils Consumption			
Fermented Foods Consumption			
Water Consumption			
Sugar Avoidance			
Processed Foods Avoidance			
Not Smoking			
Other:			

Rate Your Body Systems:

Example:	Poor	Average	Excellent
Sleep Quality		X	
Digestion			
Energy			
Immunity			
Hormone Balance			
Weight			
Brain Clarity			
Other:			
Other:			

In week 7, we'll come back and review the Living Wellness Assessment. You may be surprised at all of the changes that occur over the next six weeks.

Week 1, Day 4: Breaking the Cycle of Shame

Today we will be shedding light on some potentially deep-seeded lies about ourselves. These lies must be discussed and addressed in order to live out God's best for our lives. This process is emotional and illuminating. Be sure to give yourself adequate time and space for self-reflection on today's reading.

Feeling *shame* is believing a lie about who we are. People who live with shame often deal with low self-esteem and turn to unhealthy, life-controlling issues such as food addiction and obsessive dieting or exercising to cope with their perceived inadequacies. These unhealthy habits lead to poor choices that lead to shame, leading to more poor choices. This is the cycle of shame, which negatively affects our health in every way.

People often confuse feeling ashamed, which is a result of something we did wrong or something that was done to us, with shame.

In his book *Healing the Hurts of Your Past: A Guide to Overcoming the Pain of Shame*, F. Remy Diederich describes how "shame is rooted in the hurts of our past. How we deal with it can be the difference between staying stuck in emotional pain and rising up to become the person God created you to be." Living with shame, or believing a lie about ourselves, often procures deep, unintended consequences.

Below is an excerpt from Dawn, my friend and Living Wellness co-founder, regarding her struggle with shame:

> Shame was like carrying around giant packs of extra food on my back. I couldn't get the packs off—I would fumble through the grocery store, get angry at my mom for teaching me such terrible food habits, angry at my dad for telling me that I didn't need to learn how to cook, that was women's work, not professional women's work.

> The Living Wellness education and meditations helped me remember and heal all my old unconscious shameful patterns. Those patterns created the "I'm not good enough" or fat storage and stressful energy in my stomach. The stress and lies of shame weighed my entire body and life down. I prayed for God to shine new energy (his truth) into my stomach. The combination of God's love, a dose of education, and love from the facilitators helped me to throw off those packs of shame and extra weight off my back.

> Shame is heavy, it's uncomfortable, and it's so painful—get rid of it! Let God heal you by revealing the *truth* of who you are in him.

The number-one shame trigger for women is body image or believing the lie that we are not whole or complete because our bodies are not "perfect." The number-one shame trigger for men is being perceived as weak or inadequate. The root of shame reveals a lie regarding what we believe about ourselves. A trusted friend and mentor once told me, "God is not

[just] interested in your spiritual life; he is interested in your *whole* life!" Understanding the truth about our relationship to God changes our perspectives on life. I know that I am a daughter of God. He has received me into his family, by grace, and there is no bad thing I can do to be kicked out of his family. It's not about me; rather, my identity is found in Jesus! This knowledge allows me to examine lies I once believed about myself and replace them with God's truth.

Lies and Truth

In order to learn new habits, you must unlearn old ones. Let's look at some statements that I believe to be lies meant to keep you stuck in a cycle of sick and unhealthy. Then we will examine the corresponding truths.

Lie: God only cares about my spiritual well-being.

Truth: In the first years of Jesus's ministry, he went from city to city healing physical, mental, and spiritual maladies. If God only cares about the health of our souls, why are there so many accounts of physical healing by Jesus himself? I believe God cares about the health of our entire being, mind, body, and spirit.

Lie: I am vain if I work out and care about my physical health.

Truth: Proverbs 31:17: "She sets about her work vigorously; her arms are strong for her tasks." How can we perform the work of God if we are not physically up to the task? People who work out have more energy, sleep better, have stronger immune systems, have higher self-esteem, and are better able to manage stress. Vanity is the unhealthy love of one's outward image. Proper nutrition and exercise, on the other hand, are our best natural medicine!

Lie: I am selfish if I spend time caring for myself.

Truth: Jesus spent time away from the crowds—time away to rest and pray. He was not *always* serving people. He nourished his body, mind, and spirit, and his relationships with his father and others. Taking time to care for yourself is a gift, and it leads to your overall health and well-being.

Lie: I can't afford to eat healthily.

Truth: You can't afford *not* to eat healthily. Saying you can't afford to eat healthily is like saying you don't have time to stop for gasoline on a road trip. Let me explain. Most people who try to save money by eating cheap food do *not* ever feel satisfied and filled up, therefore eating twice as much as if they were to just eat a healthy, balanced meal in the first place. If you eat less food, you will spend the same amount as if you ate twice as much junk food, *and* you will be more satisfied because healthy food fills you up! You will pay for your health—either by investing in healthy food and exercise or by suffering from a preventable (costly) illness or injury. Choose life!

Imagine driving when your low gas light turns on. You could say, *I don't have time to stop for gas.* However, once you run out of fuel and have to call a tow truck, you're going to be out double the money than if you had pulled over and bought the gas in the first place. Invest in yourself on the front end and save yourself the cash; you'll have a much more vibrant, energetic life for the ride!

Lie: If I work out, I can eat whatever I want to.

Truth: You sure can put whatever you want to in your mouth, but if it's not nourishing to your body, there will be consequences. What you put in your body makes up your cells, your DNA—if you put toxic or even non-nourishing food in your body, you may burn off the calories, but exercise will not rid your body of all the toxins. You can't out-exercise a bad diet.

Which of the above lies do you believe? Are there others?

_____

_____

Who will you be when you break the chains of negative self-talk, low self-esteem, and self-doubt (example: a person who is free to serve others, or a person who breaks the cycle of people pleasing)?

_____

_____

_____

Make a Plan for Overcoming the Excuse Muse

She talks to each of us in different ways. What is the Excuse Muse whispering in your ear? Circle all that apply:

• I'm too busy • Temptation is too strong • I'm afraid I will fail • I'm just too tired • I'm not motivated • Bad habits are more fun • I'm distracted • I'm not worth the hassle • I want to get back at someone with my bad choices • My spouse is not worth the work it takes for me to look good • If I lose weight, people who have been nagging me to lose weight will have won

Do you have other excuses? What are they?

_____

_____

_____

_____

How do you plan to overcome these excuses?

_____

_____

_____

One way of overcoming excuses is through positive self-talk.

Practice Positive Self-Talk

You have thoughts about yourself going through your mind constantly. Part of being healthy is respecting yourself with those thoughts.

Positive self-talk is a crucial part of endurance in your wellness journey. You have an *opportunity* to be healthier; it is not a chore or a curse. You have the *ability* to make choices; you are not hopeless in your current situation. You have the *strength* to honor your body with physical activity rather than dreading another workout. Repeat these phrases:

- I get to be healthier.
- I make wise choices.
- I am strong, and I enjoy moving my body in the way it was designed.
- I am created for more than mediocre health.

Or make up your own!

If your attitude needs a boost, practice daily positive self-talk until your words become reality. And then remember to positive self-talk if you find yourself slipping back into old habits.

What does God say about you and your health? Spend time in prayer reflecting on scripture. If you are unsure of where to start, reference this list of scriptural truths.

Who We Are in Christ

I praise you because I am fearfully and wonderfully made; your works are wonderful, I know that full well. Psalms 139:14

I can do all this through him who gives me strength. Philippians 4:13

Being confident of this, that he who began a good work in you will carry it on to completion until the day of Christ Jesus. Philippians 1:6

"For I know the plans I have for you," declares the Lord, "plans to prosper you and not to harm you, plans to give you hope and a future." Jeremiah 29:11

He replied, "Because you have so little faith. Truly I tell you, if you have faith as small as a mustard seed, you can say to this mountain, 'Move from here to there,' and it will move. Nothing will be impossible for you." Matthew 17:20

So God created mankind in his own image, in the image of God he created them; male and female he created them. Genesis 1:27

For we are God's handiwork, created in Christ Jesus to do good works, which God prepared in advance for us to do. Ephesians 2:10

Make a notecard or bookmark with the truths you wrote about your health. Allow God's truth about who you are to direct your thoughts and actions. Refer to your notes daily.

Week 1, Day 5: The Root Why – Why Do You Eat?

Every twenty-eight days, your skin replaces itself. Your liver, five months. Your bones, ten years. Your body makes these new cells from the food you eat. What you eat literally becomes you.

– Dr. Biddington

"When the woman saw that the fruit of the tree was good for food and pleasing to the eye, and also desirable for gaining wisdom, she took some and ate it. She also gave some to her husband, who was with her, and he ate it" (Genesis 3:6).

Our messed-up relationship with distrusting God started in Genesis. We chose to defy God because we thought he was holding out on us. We thought there was something better to be had, something tastier, so we plucked and ate the fruit to find out for ourselves.

This original sin grieved God so deeply. Can you imagine? The one instruction he gave Adam and Eve was not to eat the fruit from *that* tree. There were consequences of their choice to disobey God: disease, decay, and even death was the result of disobedience. The act of eating the fruit itself wasn't the problem. The problem was not trusting God's best and then deliberately disobeying. It makes me so sad to think of that moment, but do you know what makes me sadder? This act of distrust and disobedience happens every day. I find myself struggling with the issue of trusting God in other areas of my life. And because the norm is to trust everyone else before God with our health, we mindlessly put unhealthy food and drink in our mouths and neglect our physical health more often than not. I'm not judging anyone's actions here; first and foremost I speak from personal experience.

Why do we eat?

Your answers may be "To fuel my body," "To give myself energy," or "Because I like the taste of food." If you're being really honest (think of the root why), you may have thought about emotional eating: boredom, stress, anxiety, mindlessness, and on and on. These are all very real reasons for why we eat. But have you recently (or ever) stopped to think about why God wants you to eat?

I remember when I began exploring such questions as: "Does God care about my physical health?" "What is the relationship between my health and my faith?" "Do I need to physically suffer all the time with pain and illness, or is there something I can (and should) do to be a better steward of my body?" The answers are so life-giving!

Why do *you* eat?

_____

_____

_____

The fourth-century BCE philosopher Socrates nailed it when he said, "Let food be thy medicine and medicine be thy food."

At some point in history we stopped relying on our natural resources and started creating chemicals in a lab to treat the complexities of our natural bodies.

Do not get me wrong: I am *not* anti-medicine. I am so grateful to live in an era where I can get emergency medical care twenty-four hours a day. One of my children recently received life-saving medicine to open her airways. I was on my knees thanking God for epinephrine that day.

There is a place for medicine.

But use your imagination for a moment. What would happen if we all started to eat to nourish our bodies, rather than to stuff them and satisfy every craving? What would happen if we made our food choices based on what we needed in a given day rather than what was handed to us through a window? Disease would decline, and our energy levels would skyrocket. Remember, your cells are made up of everything you feed them. Eating fake food will not result in vibrant health.

Eating to Nourish

I realize that this message is not going to be popular because what is required to obtain exceptional health takes grit, as author and pastor of the Willow Creek Community Church, Bill Hybels, likes to say. Transformation takes time, not pills. An abundant life takes practice, not quick fixes. Life to the fullest demands discipline and accountability, not self-reliance and a pick-yourself-up-by-your-bootstraps attitude. But that's why you're here! You have an opportunity of a lifetime. Take this opportunity to learn and reflect on your health and be blessed!

Friends, the road toward better health is challenging, *but it is full of life*. Trust God with your journey. God knows what you need. And guess what? If you go to him openly, he will reveal what you need. Have patience and endurance. You are worth exceptional health.

So why *should* you eat?

_____

_____

_____

What in your health will change when you *eat to nourish* your body?

_____

Week 1, Day 6: What Should You Eat?

Now knowing why we should eat—to nourish our body rather than to simply fill a void—let's focus on *what* we should eat.

The FOSS Health Continuum Chart is shown below. I developed this chart after working with individuals and families to "health-up" their pantries. Rather than asking, *Is this food good or bad?*, ask yourself, *Is this my best option in this circumstance?*

Start with the chart below when you're ready to transform your pantry and your health.

FOSS (Flour, Oil, Sugar, and Salt) Continuum Chart

Even the healthiest people usually don't eat unprocessed food 100 percent of the time. Your goal is to slowly move away from eating foods in the left column and move toward eating unprocessed foods. Some foods and beverages may be easy and painless for you to switch out; some may take a lifetime. Remember your health is a journey. This chart is a guide to help you make the best decisions in any given situation, not a diet plan for strict adherence. A lifetime of small changes in the right direction will lead to consistently better health.

FOSS	Processed Food (Toxic)–Avoid	Less Processed (Some Health Benefits)	Unprocessed (Nourishing)– Enjoy in Moderation	Enjoy with Reckless Abandon
Flour & Grains	Enriched flour Bleached flour Bulgur White flour products Puffed grain products, such as rice cakes Factory-made modern soy foods Soybeans, unless used for making fermented foods like natto Soybean sprouting seeds and sprouts Alfalfa seeds and sprouts	100 percent whole grains Unsoaked granola Dried beans and lentils Unsoaked whole-grain rice Canned beans Buckwheat, corn, and brown rice pasta Organic white rice	Soaked and/or sprouted grains; fermented grains, such as sourdough Organic dried beans and lentils Soaked and/or sprouted 100 percent whole grains and whole-grain breakfast cereals that must be cooked Wild rice Organic popcorn (to pop at home) Organic sprouting seeds except alfalfa and soybean	Nothing except the love of Jesus!

Your goal is to slowly move away from eating foods in the left column and move toward eating unprocessed foods.

FOSS	Processed Food (Toxic)–Avoid	Less Processed (Some Health Benefits)	Unprocessed (Nourishing)– Enjoy in Moderation	Enjoy with Reckless Abandon
Oils & Fats	Partially hydrogenated oils Most commercial vegetable oils, including cottonseed, soy, corn, canola, rice bran, hemp, and grapeseed oils All margarines, spreads, and partially hydrogenated vegetable shortenings	Pasteurized grass-fed butter Cold-pressed or expeller-pressed sesame, sunflower, peanut, macadamia, avocado, almond, walnut, pecan, pistachio, hazelnut, pumpkin seed, and high-oleic safflower oils in small amounts Refined palm oil Refined coconut oil Extra-virgin olive oil Cold-pressed flaxseed oil	Raw grass-fed butter, organic cold-pressed flaxseed oil, extra-virgin sesame oil, red palm oil Organic extra-virgin olive oil Organic cold-pressed macadamia, avocado, almond, high-oleic sunflower, and high-oleic safflower oils Organic unrefined virgin coconut oil Unrefined organic palm oil Fat and lard from pigs allowed to graze Tallow and suet from grass-fed cows and sheep Poultry fat from pastured poultry	It's a fallacy that you can eat endless amounts of anything.
Sugar	White sugar, corn syrup, high fructose corn syrup, yacon syrup, imitation syrups, stevia extracts (powder) Artificial sweeteners, such as sucralose (Splenda) and aspartame (NutraSweet and Equal); sugar alcohols, such as xylitol	Organic sugar in the raw Organic jams Heated honey Brown rice syrup Organic blue agave Jams made with organic sugar Concentrated fruit juices Organic liquid stevia	Organic fruit Organic natural sweeteners, such as molasses, green stevia leaves and green stevia powder, dehydrated sugar cane juice, malt syrups, coconut sugar, palm sugar, date sugar, and sorghum syrup Maple syrup, maple sugar Raw honey, preferably unfiltered	The key to long-term health success is:
Salt	Table salt, sodium nitrite, sodium nitrate Monosodium glutamate (MSG)	Kosher salt Commercial sea salt	Unrefined mineral salt, such as Celtic sea salt or pink Himalayan (generally, salt should have a color)	MODERATION

What do you call a really old rock? (Answer: A fossil.) What will you get if you don't update your FOSS? (Answer: You get ill.) Don't become a fossil before it's your time, friend! ☺

Another helpful tool when selecting *what to eat* is the Environmental Working Group's (EWG) Guide to Pesticides in Produce. I often take and use this chart at the grocery store, especially when shopping with a budget. The Dirty Dozen have been shown to contain high amounts of pesticides, even after being washed and peeled. Whereas, the Clean Fifteen have been found to have little to no pesticides after being washed and peeled.

2016 EWG Shopper's Guide to Pesticides in Produce

Dirty Dozen (always buy organic)	Clean Fifteen (OK to eat nonorganic)
Strawberries	Avocados
Apples	Sweet Corn*
Nectarines	Pineapple
Peaches	Cabbage
Celery	Sweet peas–frozen
Grapes	Onions
Cherries	Asparagus
Spinach	Mangoes
Tomatoes	Papayas*
Sweet bell peppers	Kiwi
Cherry tomatoes	Eggplant
Cucumbers	Honeydew melon
	Grapefruit
	Cantaloupe
	Cauliflower

*Most sweet corn, papaya, and summer squash sold in the United States are produced from genetically engineered (GE) seeds. The EWG says to "buy organic varieties of these crops if you want to avoid GE produce."

> Eating diet food is like eating a hologram—there's nothing there!

Physical and Spiritual Satisfaction

If the food you eat does not nourish you (think white bread or candy), your body is going to continue to signal hunger because you did not achieve the satisfaction from nutrients. This is why so many people on diets are hungry all the time and why they don't achieve long-term success. Dieters eat diet food containing few real nutrients and/or healthy fat, and the body says, "I can taste something, but there's no substance." Eating diet food is like eating a hologram—there's nothing there! Our bodies crave nutrients, not mere calories.

Nourishing your body is much like nourishing your spirit. We all have a God-sized hole in our hearts. If we don't recognize that the longing is for a relationship with God, we will try to fill that void with other things: food, shopping, alcohol, friends, spouse, thrills, and the like. If we keep transferring our longings from one vice, addiction, or life-controlling issue to another, our souls will remain unsatisfied. Whether we recognize it or not, our souls all long for a deep relationship with God, and only he can fill that spot in our hearts.

How Much Fuel Does Your Body Need?

What happens when you try to fill a water balloon with more water than it can handle? Either the water spills out or the balloon bursts! The amount of water you put in depends on the size of the balloon. The fat cells in your body react much the same way.

At five-foot, three-inches tall, do you think I need to consume the same amount of food as my six-foot-one husband? No! If I did, I would probably double in size (and not in the tall way). Most people who have access to an abundance of food, especially processed food, overeat. Why? People overeat for a variety of reasons: mindlessness, stress, emotions, comfort, hunger, and the list goes on. The most common reason for overeating is that we don't consistently eat to nourish our bodies.

Do you find yourself overeating? Why?

_____

_____

_____

_____

_____

_____

_____

_____

Let's take a look at the benefits *inside the body* when we eat for nourishment.

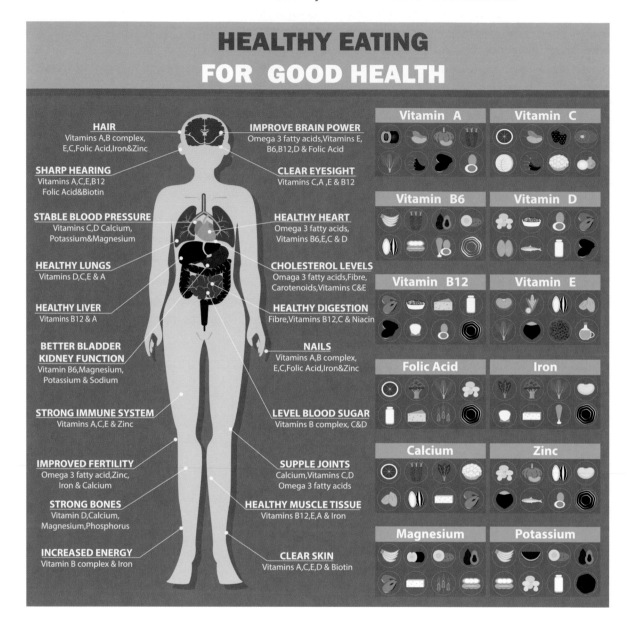

To nourish all the cells and systems of your body, you need macronutrients (protein, carbs, and fat), micronutrients (vitamins and minerals), water, and healthy bacteria to maintain proper gut balance. Authors Dr. Natasha Campbell-McBride, MD, and researcher Westin A. Price lay out guidelines on how to properly nourish the body that include more detail than the government's simplistic MyPlate. Using these experts' guidelines, your three main meals may look something like this:

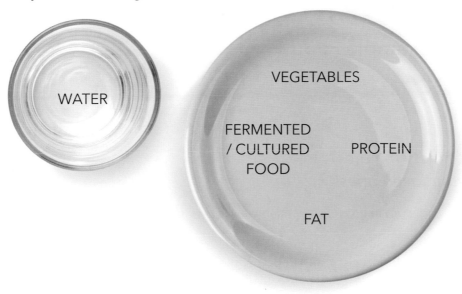

Your snacks may look something like this:

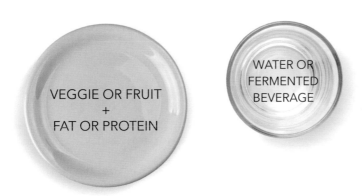

Now you may be asking, *"Where is the dairy in this meal plan?"* I'm a lover of raw milk, hard cheeses, and homemade yogurt, but due to modern processing, many people do not digest dairy well. And since dairy is not an essential need for our bodies, I leave it up to you to decide. How well do you feel after eating diary? Do you have asthma, allergies, or skin rashes? If so, you may want to avoid dairy for at least three weeks to see if your symptoms improve. Once your nutrition is squeaky clean and your gut is healed, you'll have a really good sense for what your body wants and needs and what it does not. This process takes a little time. Be patient.

Food Prep

Food preparation saves you time and money. In most cases, when you plan and prep your food in advance rather than resorting to fast food, gas station snacks, or even going to a reasonably nice restaurant, you will be much more nourished with your own, whole foods. Keeping staples on hand and throwing together a salad is quicker than ordering takeout.

Ashley's Weekly Example Food-Prep Routine

Below is an example of my weekly prep routine. *If I don't have time to prep all at once,* I break the list up throughout the week as my schedule allows:

Prep Time: About ninety minutes
Serves: You and your loved ones!

- [ ] Wash fruits; slice and store in fridge, if applicable (always wash your produce, even if it has a peel)

- [ ] Wash vegetables like carrots, celery, and peppers; slice and store in resealable baggies or glass containers in the fridge (great alternative to chips—try with salsa, hummus, or guacamole)

- [ ] Bake or boil eggs (protein-rich, on-the-go snack—be sure to wash—remember, salmonella is on the outside of the egg)

- [ ] Peel ripe bananas; store and freeze (for smoothies, baking, or to eat frozen—great alternative to ice cream!)

- [ ] Soak seeds, nuts, beans, and grains (soaking removes antinutrients); then dehydrate or cook

- [ ] Make homemade trail mix from your last batch of soaked and dehydrated nuts, seeds, and fruit (nutrient-rich, on-the-go snack)

- [ ] Make or bottle kombucha (fermented food) —instructions in Appendix A

- [ ] Make bone broth—(It's a great base for soup, rice, grains, pasta, and vegetables. Some people even drink it warm, straight from a mug)—instructions in Appendix A

- [ ] Make or feed sourdough starter—recipe in week 6 (sourdough must be cared for daily or placed in fridge to keep fresh)

- [ ] Put something in the slow cooker (a roast, a chicken, beans, or rice—slow cooker meals are perfect for on-the-go people—add a veggie and you've got a meal)

How will you incorporate food prep into your weekly routine to help you eat better?

Be specific.

_____

_____

_____

_____

_____

What day(s) will you shop?

_____

_____

_____

_____

_____

What day(s) will you meal-prep?

_____

_____

_____

_____

What staples will you have on hand for quick meals and snacks?

_____

_____

_____

_____

_____

Week 1, Day 7: Recap & Reflect

Welcome to the end of week 1. At the end of each week, you will be recapping important concepts and highlights. The recap will be followed by a time for reflection. Feel free to read this section first to get a complete picture of the week before you begin.

- *Living Wellness for Growth Groups* gives you the tools and resources to be a healthier version of yourself. You have the choice and ability to step into that journey.

- Count calories in a wellness journal. People who journal are more successful.

- Physical discipline is just as important as spiritual discipline. You are a reflection of God—he wants the best for your life.

- God knows what is best for you, and he wants what is best for your health. Sometimes this requires sacrifice or change, but trust that God is good. Listen to the promptings he is giving you and make the necessary changes.

- God cares about your whole self—mind, body, and spirit.

- Feeling ashamed is a result of something we did wrong or something that was done to us. Feeling *shame* is believing a lie about who we are. Shame keeps us stuck in destructive patterns. Ask God to reveal the lies you believe about yourself and your body and then ask God to heal them and replace them with his truths.

- Your motivations (your root why) will guide your thoughts and your actions (why you eat and exercise).

- Your plate should be full of vegetables, protein, healthy fat, and small servings of fruit and fermented foods. Practice eating to nourish your body, slow down, and always give thanks! Avoid processed foods. Use the FOSS chart in Appendix D when grocery shopping and reading labels.

Reflection

1. Look back at your health goal brainstorm from day 1. Choose the number one Living Wellness Growth Group health goal you want to accomplish in the next seven weeks.

2. Write your goal here as a SMART goal:

_____

_____

_____

_____

_____

3. Practice the root why exercise with your health goal:

_____

_____

Why is this a goal?

_____

_____

Why?

_____

_____

Why?

_____

_____

Why?

_____

_____

4. Use your weekly action steps as objectives to help you achieve this goal.

5. What could potentially get in the way of you achieving this goal?

_____

_____

6. How can you overcome these challenges?

_____

_____

As you gain knowledge about yourself and health, another goal may rise to the surface. Use the space provided to explore these new goals.

Living Wellness Growth Group Health Goal:

_____

_____

Why?

_____

_____

Why?

_____

_____

Why?

_____

_____

1. Use your weekly action steps as objectives to help you achieve this goal.

_____

_____

_____

2. What could potentially get in the way of you achieving this goal?

_____

_____

_____

3. How can you overcome these challenges?

_____

_____

Living Wellness Growth Group Health Goal:

_____

_____

Why?

_____

_____

Why?

_____

_____

Why?

_____

_____

1. Use your weekly action steps as objectives to help you achieve this goal.

_____

_____

2. What could potentially get in the way of you achieving this goal?

_____

_____

3. How can you overcome these challenges?

_____

_____

Well done on completing your first week!

Reflection Notes:

_____

_____

_____

_____

_____

_____

_____

_____

_____

_____

_____

_____

_____

_____

_____

_____

_____

_____

_____

_____

_____

_____

_____

_____

_____

_____

_____

_____

_____

_____

_____

_____

_____

_____

_____

_____

_____

_____

_____

_____

_____

_____

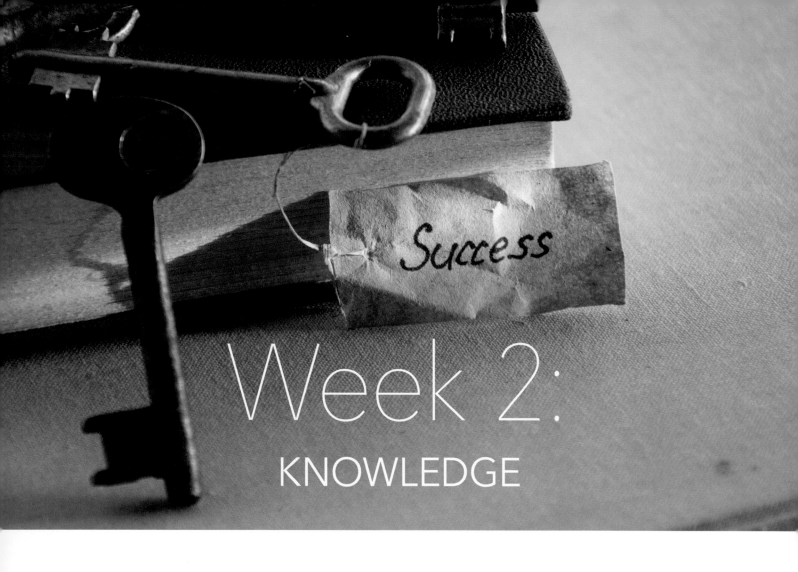

Week 2:
KNOWLEDGE

This week is all about gaining knowledge (one of the five keys to success) about the inner workings of our bodies and practicing what we learn.

Perhaps you have heard the phrase *knowledge is power*. When you have the knowledge about what foods nourish and what foods harm your body, you have the opportunity to take your health into your own hands. When you have the knowledge of how to work out and stretch properly, you can exercise confidently. When you have the knowledge that God cares about your health and well-being, you can make decisions that positively impact the health of your whole self. Arm yourself with knowledge this week.

> **But until a person can say deeply and honestly, "I am what I am today because of the choices I made yesterday," that person cannot say, "I choose otherwise."**
>
> —Stephen R. Covey

Week 2 Action Steps

Number one health goal: _____ *Goal Accomplished!* ☐

Accountability

Record your **strength** workouts in the *Living Wellness Journal*;

weekly goal:_____ _____ (number of days) (minutes per day) ☐

    Partner's goal: _____ _____ (number of days) (minutes per day)

Record your **cardio** workouts in the *Living Wellness Journal*;

weekly goal:_____ _____ (number of days) (minutes per day) ☐

    Partner's goal: _____ _____ (number of days) (minutes per day)

Your **nutrition** goal (Remember the SMART goals) _____ ☐

    Partner's goal: _____ _____

Check in with your partner daily. ☐ ☐ ☐ ☐ ☐ ☐ ☐

Knowledge

Read and fill out all questions in this book *prior* to the next meeting. ☐

Mindfulness

Write about how you feel after a workout: _____ ☐

Inspiration

How will you nourish your spiritual health this week (i.e. prayer, reading scripture, church community, Christian conference, listening to a faith-based broadcast, acts of service, fasting, tithing, your relationship with God)?

_____ ☐

Motivation

What motivated you to begin your journey toward living a healthier lifestyle?

_____ ☐

Living Wellness Week 2 Exercise

Add this core exercise to your existing strength training routine.

Leg Lifts

Lie on your back and place your hands under your low back. Bend your knees and lift them straight in the air. Exhale and pull your belly button into your spine as you slowly lower your bent legs. Lower until your back can no longer maintain a flat posture with your back against the ground. Alternate lifting your legs.

For Option II, perform the leg lifts with straight legs with both legs at a time.

Repeat for 16 to 20 reps. Repeat as time permits. Practice this exercise every other day. Remember to stretch after your workout.

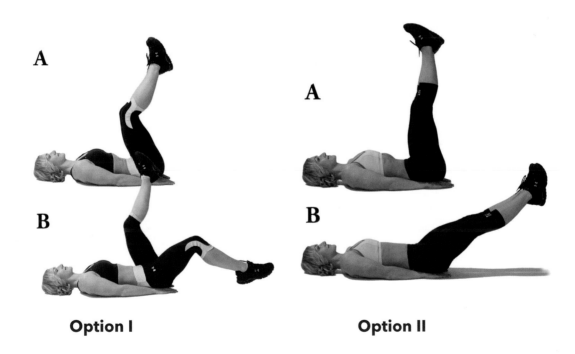

Option I   **Option II**

Looking Ahead

This week you will learn about ingredients to avoid, proper protein and produce amounts and choices, and how to eat well on every budget.

Week 2, Day 2: Metabolism

Years ago, when I first started talking about the metabolism, I used to describe it as a woodstove: throw a log on to get it started and then feed it before it burns out. Simple, right? In some regards, this does describe the importance of eating regularly throughout the day, rather than skipping meals and eating all at once. But your metabolism is so much more complex. Your metabolism is more like the inner workings of a city, controlling the flow of processes, hormones, and systems within your body.

What Is the Function of Your Metabolism?

The chemistry behind your metabolism is complicated. Think of your metabolism as the stoplights and law enforcement in a city, carefully regulating the flow of traffic to maintain peace, much like your body chemistry (metabolism) constantly regulating chemicals and hormones to maintain balance. According to an article from the Mayo Clinic staff (2014), your metabolism is responsible for breaking down, digesting, absorbing, transporting, and storing or burning the food you consume (calories). There are many moving parts in an efficient traffic flow and in a healthy metabolism.

It's easy to blame weight gain on a slow metabolism as a result of age or genetics, but in reality, the speed or rate that you burn calories has more to do with what you eat and how often you exercise. Your metabolism is a chemistry lab, not a drag race. Unless you have a metabolic disorder, *weight gain is a result of consuming more and/or the wrong kind of calories than your body needs—usually because the calories we consume are void of nutritional value, causing you to eat more.*

We may feel like our metabolisms keep us looking to sugar for energy to get up and go, *but usually the sugar we eat damages the inner workings of our metabolisms.* Consuming added sugar turns on the *red light* for burning fat as fuel. But healthy fats, like avocados, turn on the *green light* for burning fat as fuel. The foods we eat, how often we eat, how much water we drink, how much muscle we have, how much sleep we get, and how often we exercise affect the flow of our metabolisms.

You can improve the chemistry of your metabolism *today.* You can make small, effective changes that *will* impact how you look and feel instantly. Eventually, your body composition will reflect your new choices.

Five Ways to Boost Your Metabolism Right Now!

1. **Move your body every day!** Muscle is one of the most important factors in the health of your metabolism (the number of calories your body burns in movement *and* at rest each and every day). *The more muscle you have, the more fuel you burn.* Muscle burns ten times more calories than other tissue. *One pound of body fat burns five calories in twenty-four hours compared to one pound of muscle that burns fifty calories per day,*

each and every day! Cardio exercise boosts your metabolism for several hours after your workout. In comparison, muscle mass raises your metabolism *all day, every day*, because muscle burns fat all day long! Does strength training sound more attractive now? Your lean muscle mass is one of the most significant factors in your metabolic rate. Muscle burns body fat! Celebrate! The Living Wellness workout you are practicing throughout these eight weeks is a strength-training, muscle-building workout!

2. **Eat breakfast** and small meals every three to four hours. You would not expect your vehicle to run without fuel, and you should not expect your body to, either. Breakfast is meant to *break the fast*. You will feel your best when you go to bed with an empty stomach and your body is ready to eat and be energized in the morning. You should eat something healthy within one hour of waking. If breakfast upsets your stomach, try something with less acid (an egg rather than orange juice, for example). After breakfast, you should eat small meals or snacks every three to four hours—a couple of hundred calories each depending on your caloric needs.

3. **Water, water, water**. One study published in the *Journal of Clinical Endocrinology and Metabolism* reports that drinking seventeen ounces of water (preferably filtered) in one sitting increases metabolic rate by 30 percent! Your body uses calories to process water. Remember, you should be drinking approximately half of your ideal body weight in ounces every day. In addition to boosting your metabolism, water is also responsible for bringing nutrients into and removing waste from every cell. Water also aids in digestion, balances body fluids, helps you feel full, keeps your muscles energized, keeps your skin elastic, and flushes your kidneys and liver. Imagine putting yesterday's lunch in a blender. How would your blender sound when you turned it on? Now, imagine adding 20 ounces of water to the blender—the contents would digest better. Our stomachs and our digestive tracts need water, as does every cell in our bodies.

4. **Sleep.** The US Department of Health and Human Services recommends adults need about seven to eight hours, teens need at least nine hours, children need ten to twelve hours, and babies need sixteen to eighteen hours of sleep every day. Not only is getting adequate sleep a necessity, it has a variety of health benefits:

   - You will be less likely to get sick.
   - You lower your risk of high blood pressure and diabetes.
   - You boost your brainpower and your mood.

For Better Sleep (Lawrence Epstein, MD):

- Keep a regular sleep/ wake schedule.

- Develop a pre-sleep routine.

- Reserve the bedroom for sleep and intimacy.

- Practice daily exercise to burn off extra energy.

- Maintain a healthy diet.

- Do not drink to excess or smoke.

Circle the points you can work on to start sleeping better.

- You think more clearly and do better in school and at work.

- You make better decisions and avoid injuries; sleepy drivers cause thousands of car crashes every year.

- You will be more likely to attain and maintain a healthy weight.

I don't talk much more about the benefits of sleep throughout this study. But let me assure you, sleep is one of the greatest assets you have to being healthy and avoiding premature aging. I strongly encourage you to create a healthy environment for sleeping. Set a bedtime routine. Make sure you have a good mattress, pillows, and sheets. Where else do you spend so much time in your life? Perhaps only your workplace rivals the bedroom if you work outside the home. Get good sleep. Fight for good sleep. Make it a priority and your health, energy, and mood will improve.

5. **Your plate**. Your body requires balanced nutrition in order to function properly. Eating processed carbohydrates, such as muffins, hamburger buns, crackers, white pasta, candy, and pizza crust feeds bad bacteria in your gut, which in turn throws off the balance in your body and messes up your metabolism! Intestines and bowels filled with too many processed foods get clogged, inflamed, and damaged. To maintain a healthy metabolism, our plates should be filled with vegetables, healthy fat, protein, fermented food, and a limited amount of fruit.

A Toxic Metabolism

As previously stated, the cells of your body are largely made up of what you feed them. You are what you eat! Likewise, your metabolism functions on everything you eat. If you are consistently overeating processed food and toxins, your body is producing more chemicals to process and break down the toxins. Toxins put stress on every organ in your body. For example, if you consistently ingest too much synthetic salt (table salt), your heart must work extra hard to eliminate the extra salt from the body, stressing it. Too much of anything is tantamount to not enough.

What negative habit is diminishing the effectiveness of your metabolism?

_____

_____

_____

What changes will you make to improve the health of your metabolism today?

_____

_____

How will you feel when your metabolism is improved?

_____

_____

_____

Not enough nourishment, such as a fat-free diet (which is often laden with extra sugar and chemicals), is just as damaging to the metabolism as overeating. We eat because we like the taste of food. Manufacturers know this. They study your preferences and base their careers on producing cheap, delicious food. Often this results in adding pernicious chemicals to your food to hyperexcite your taste buds.

Reading labels is an essential part of recognizing food as nourishment because, while chemical additives may excite your taste buds, they do not love and honor your DNA. On the contrary, chemical additives break down body functions and destroy our DNA and put us at risk for a whole host of diseases (look up *epigenetics* if you're interested in reading more about food and DNA).

When you shop, take the time to read labels. Start with the *ingredients* list rather than the *nutrition facts*. When you read the ingredients list, you will be able to determine if the product contains real food as opposed to a chemical look-alike. The ingredients appear in order of relative quantity; if sugar is the first item on the list, there is more sugar in the food or beverage than any other ingredient. Bring the Ingredients to Avoid section (in the next section) and the FOSS Chart to the grocery store and check the ingredients against both lists. It may seem cumbersome to read every label in the store, but I promise it is worth your time. You will soon be able to quickly recognize whole foods. You will feel better, look better, have more energy, and have fewer toxins in your body. And the more you're aware of labels, the easier shopping gets. You will know which brands have consistently clean(er) ingredients and which brands go the cheaper, chemical, and processed route.

> *Not enough nourishment, such as a fat-free diet (which is often laden with extra sugar and chemicals), is just as damaging to the metabolism as overeating.*

Week 2, Day 3: Ingredients to Avoid

Today we continue to gain knowledge as we examine common toxic ingredients found in most processed and packaged foods. Use this list to recognize harmful foods as you shop.

Harmful Preservatives

I say *harmful* because some forms of preserving food are not damaging. For example, when you put your grapes in the freezer, this will preserve them, but it will not harm the food in the process.

Partially hydrogenated oil

This is a harmful preservative that adds hydrogen to the oil at a high heat. According to the Mayo Clinic, this process of adding hydrogen to preserve the oil negatively throws off the balance of your cholesterol (LDL/HDL) among a long list of terrible health implications that we will tackle in week 5. Have you ever seen a fast-food burger that was (purposefully) left out in a doctor's office for years and it did not look any different from how it did when it was bought? Think about how it looks inside your body. The substance does not effortlessly break down because of the massive number of preservatives in the burger. No meat, cheese, or carbohydrate should be able to sit out in the open without decomposing. Avoid putting anything in your body that is pumped with *embalming-like oil*.

I tell my clients to think about partially hydrogenated oils like liquid glue added to the oil. It sticks to your body and does not easily break down. Have you ever quit eating fast food for a period of time and then caved in and eaten a fast-food cheeseburger and fries or some variety of fried food? That stomachache you got after eating was the food sitting in your stomach like a magnetic lump of glue, attracting bad bacteria. Ugh. It's no wonder we have so many stomach problems. Avoid preservatives and you will reduce your stomach complications.

BHA and BHT

Otherwise known as butylated hydroxyanisole and butylated hydroxytoluene. Similar to partially hydrogenated oils, these preservatives keep the last leftover perishable nutrients in highly processed oils in foods from going rancid. They do not belong in food because your body does not recognize the chemicals. Along with highly processed oils, unrecognizable chemicals are suggested to increase your chances of getting cancer.

Sodium benzoate, nitrates and nitrites, sulfates, potassium bromate—like all the chemicals above, they do not belong in your body, and they should be avoided as much as possible.

There are whole books dedicated to the harmful effects of preservatives in our foods. The key is to look for whole-food recipes that you can prepare yourself and then preserve naturally. Limit your intake of packaged foods as meals and snacks. Balanced eating does not have to be all or nothing. Real plants and animal foods are not evil. The more we are mindful of what we put in our bodies, the better we will look and feel. *You are worth more than mediocre ingredients!*

Flavor Enhancers

Monosodium glutamate (MSG)

MSG is a food additive that has no purpose other than to enhance the flavor of food and get you addicted. MSG is found in some soy sauces, chips, frozen vegetable mixes, seasonings, soups, salad dressings, and packaged foods. MSG is a thyroid killer, a metabolic murderer, and a brain-sensory thief, an all-around thug. Need I say more? Read labels.

Artificial sweeteners (aspartame and sucralose [Splenda])

The problem with artificial, zero-calorie sweeteners is not necessarily in the chemicals themselves but in the damage they do to our intestines, brains, and hormones once they are in the body. Check your coffee creamer. This is a perfect place for flavor enhancers to hide! Replace chemical sweeteners with real ingredients, such as honey or real maple syrup.

Enriched Grains

This is one of the most misleading ingredients I have found on the market. The word *enriched* sounds like a positive description, right? I am sorry to disappoint, but in the context of grains, the "enriching" process leaves the product impoverished.

Imagine taking a most precious real pearl necklace and ripping all the pearls off and throwing them away. Then, imagine cutting out pictures of pearls from paper and gluing them on the strand. You would look at the final product and say *something is wrong here. This is a fake!* Most grains in America experience a similar affect in the bleaching and enriching process.

Whole kernels of wheat, rice, oat, cornmeal, or barley are rich in nutrients such as fiber, B vitamins, iron, folate, calcium, phosphorus, zinc, and copper. Your body (and brain) needs these nutrients to maintain a healthy body.

When grains are processed, they are stripped of many of these nutrients and then bleached to create a color and texture that manufacturers want us to enjoy. The problem is that when manufacturers realize the end product is not much more than Play-Doh, they enrich the substance with synthetic vitamins, much like the paper cut-out version of our pretend pearl necklace. Original, *essential* nutrients, such as fiber and B vitamins, are thrown away in the process.

When we consume enriched breads, muffins, bagels, and pasta, we are not receiving the natural forms of these important vitamins that help balance our brains and boost our moods.

Fiber is another nutrient that is not adequately replaced in the enriching process. Fiber cleanses the blood and bowels, absorbing and eliminating toxins and improving the function of your colon. We need these natural nutrients, not from processed enriched foods but from real, whole foods!

What processed foods do you have a difficult time saying "no" to?

_____

_____

_____

What unprocessed foods could replace these non-foods?

_____

_____

_____

Artificial Colors

Pause. Any time you read the word *artificial*, think, *Do I want any artificial additives in my body?* The answer should be *no*, but some are necessary (like a life-saving drug) and some are not (like artificial colors).

If you see the name of the color and a number in the ingredients, the color is artificial (FD&C Yellow 5, for example). Imagine sticking a crayon up into your brain and trying to function. You would definitely have some attention challenges with Yellow 5 in the middle of your cerebellum.

Look at a 2009 quote from Columbia and Harvard Universities on mental health studies:

"Their analysis of fifteen trials evaluating the impact of artificial food coloring suggests that removing these agents from the diets of children with ADHD would be about one-third to one-half as effective as treatment with methylphenidate (Ritalin)."

This research is suggesting that by cutting out artificial colors, children with ADHD will have one-third to one-half fewer symptoms! *This study should be a wake-up call for all of us.* Artificial colors are not healthy for our brains. This is just one small piece of the brain puzzle. The article goes on to explain what is missing from our daily nutrient intake—omega-3s and other essential vitamins and minerals—and how those too play a vital role in our (and our children's) mental health.

In addition to brain problems, artificial colors have been linked to fatigue, allergic reactions, skin rashes, asthma, and headaches. Be more aware of what you are putting into your body and how it affects your health. You are not a victim. You have options. You can make a difference in how you and your family members look and feel by taking the time to think about what goes into your mouths.

Are you willing to forgo candy that is colored artificially and make a commitment not to feed it to children? How about birthday cake? Do you know anyone who makes and colors cakes naturally?

The Good News

Regardless of what you have been consuming or how long you have been consuming it, you can make small changes in what you eat that will have an *immediate and lasting effect* on the health of your body, mind, and spirit. You were made for more than mediocre nutrition. You were made for exceptional health.

Equipped with this knowledge, continue reading labels this week.

Week 2, Day 4: Digestion

Why are we talking about digestion in this health book? Doesn't digestion happen on its own? Think about a small creek with a beaver dam running through it. The water flows on its own through the creek, but it would flow a lot better if we were proactive and cleared out that dam! Our bodies will get food from one end to the other without our thinking about it, but when we take the time to support our digestion, the response is so pleasant!

Chew Your Food

Contrary to popular belief, digestion begins in your mouth! Properly chewing your food makes it much easier for your body to break it down, absorb the food, and use it for nourishment. Next time you bite a piece of food, *count how many chews it takes you before you swallow.* See if you can slow down and chew the next bite even more. You will be better able to break down and absorb your food when it's in smaller (nearly liquid) pieces rather than big chunks.

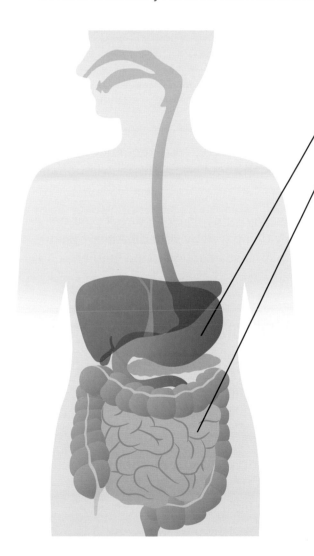

Do you know how digestion works?

After you thoroughly chew and swallow your food, it goes to the **stomach**.

Digestion: Food is broken down into tiny nutrients in the stomach.

Absorption: The nutrients are absorbed into the bloodstream from the small intestine.

Metabolism: After the nutrients are absorbed into the bloodstream, they travel to all cells in the body.

Rest While You Digest

Do you remember when your mom used to say, "No swimming for thirty minutes after you eat"? The suggestion was given to avoid drowning in the water due to cramping—because your body needs to digest food after you eat! This applies to more than just swimming (where we could drown).

One key aspect that is missing in the above process of digestion is resting—or at least relaxing. When we eat in a hurry, when we are stressed, or even while holding a grudge, the body kicks out adrenaline and other stress hormones like cortisol that make nutrient absorption difficult. When your body does not absorb the nutrients, it goes on craving more food, making you want to eat more than you actually need. If you are spending the time and money to eat healthy food, *be sure to eat mindfully, slow down, and relax while you eat* and digest so that your body gets the benefit of that healthy food!

We're Going to Talk About *What*?!

Bristol Stool Chart		
Type 1		Separate hard lumps; very constipated
Type 2		Lumpy and sausage-like; slightly constipated
Type 3		Sausage-shaped with cracks on the surface; healthy
Type 4		Sausage- or snake-like, smooth and soft; healthy
Type 5		Soft blobs with clear-cut edges; lacking fiber
Type 6		Fluffy pieces with mushy edges; inflammation
Type 7		Watery, entirely liquid; inflammation

The health of your gut can be monitored by examining your stool—the frequency and the shape and texture of your bowel movements. Yes, I'm talking about poop. This is an important indicator of your health!

In general, you should have at least one to three bowel movements every day. If your daily bowel movement is type 3 or type 4, you are probably doing well by your digestive system. If you are consistently having any other type of stool, pay close attention to the readings and discussion around digestion.

Tips to Get You Started: Improve Your Digestion Today

- Start your day with a probiotic-rich food such as yogurt or kombucha
- Drink half of your ideal body weight in ounces of filtered water every day
- Chew your food thoroughly
- Rest while you digest
- Monitor your stool and take note on which kinds of food impact your stool type
- Eat plenty of colorful vegetables to get enough fiber (see week 5, day 2)
- Consume three small servings of fermented foods daily (see week 6)

What type of stool do you usually have?

_____

_____

_____

How will you commit to improving your digestion? Reflect on some things that may be holding up your digestion; physical, emotional, or spiritual (i.e. stress, holding a grudge, or speed eating).

_____

_____

_____

_____

_____

_____

_____

_____

_____

_____

_____

_____

Week 2, Day 5: Macronutrient – Protein

Did you know? Protein rebuilds and repairs all cells, not just muscle cells.

Protein has been a hot topic on the weight management stage since the Atkins diet. What is the big deal with protein? Protein is one of three macronutrients your body needs to survive. Consuming a variety of protein is vital to exceptional health. A lack of protein causes malnourishment, atrophy or muscle loss, failure to grow, a weakened immune system, and weakened vital organs (the heart and respiratory system).

Likewise, getting too much protein without adequate water intake may have health risks as well. Breaking down and absorbing protein creates more waste than carbohydrates or fat, so if you are not consuming enough water, the process of eliminating the excess waste from your body may stress your liver or kidneys.

Two fundamentals to proper protein digestion include:

1. Eating enough quality and variety of protein.

2. Drinking at least half of your ideal body weight in ounces of water every day.

Protein:

- Rebuilds and repairs damaged cells resulting from the environment, working out, and illness
- Uses more calories to process, break down, and digest food over fat or carbohydrates. For example, it takes more energy to crush rock than to crush Play-Doh. Your body uses more energy to digest protein, creating more of a calorie deficit.
- Keeps you feeling fuller longer after meals and snacks
- Regulates moodiness
- Regulates blood sugar levels and hormones
- Boosts the immune system

How Much Protein Is Just Right?

Protein needs vary from person to person. Generally speaking, an adult should consume a minimum of 0.8 grams of protein per kilogram of body weight, which is about eight grams of protein for every twenty pounds of body weight. Competitive athletes need at least 1.2 grams of protein per kilogram of body weight.

Getting Personal

What is the daily minimum recommendation of protein based on your current weight? (Divide your body weight by 20 and then multiply that by 8)

(_____ / 20) = _____ × 8 = _____ grams (weight)

If you are an adult, use the recommendation based on your weight.

For children, a minimum recommendation of protein is broken down by age.

Recommended Dietary Allowance of Protein for Children

Age Groups	Grams of Protein Needed Per Day
Children ages 1–3	13
Children ages 4–8	19
Children ages 9–13	34
Girls ages 14–18	46
Boys ages 14–18	52

I do not consistently count grams of protein for my children. Because they consume a variety of protein at every meal and snack, they receive adequate amounts. However, if you have a picky eater or a child with food sensitivities, you may want to count grams for a few days to ensure adequate amounts. If you realize your child is not consuming enough protein, try to increase his or her intake naturally. If your child is still not consuming enough, talk to your health care provider about your options for increasing protein intake with a supplement or shake.

If you work out several hours per week, you may need more protein to maintain, rebuild, and repair muscle and cell damage, which is a natural and healthy product of exercise. Muscle breakdown and repair allows your muscles to grow stronger. Be sure to check with your doctor before altering your nutrition beyond what is recommended.

Your body is better able to absorb protein at certain times during the day. Be sure to consume one serving of protein with one serving of a carbohydrate within one hour after your workout for optimal nutrient uptake. Let's look at some examples of postexercise meals and snacks for optimal protein absorption.

Good Sources of Protein

- Preservative-free meat, free-range poultry, and fish (wild-caught when available)
- Legumes (dry beans and peas, soaked and then cooked)
- Eggs (from free-range, organic-fed chickens when available)
- Nuts and seeds (raw or soaked is better than baked or roasted)
- Milk and milk products (raw, from organic, grass-fed animals when available)
- 100 percent whole grains, some vegetables, and some fruits (all of these provide only small amounts of protein relative to animal sources)

Why don't I have protein bars and shakes listed here? Most protein bars and shakes are loaded with processed oils, sugars, salt, and preservatives. Read labels and use the FOSS chart when choosing a protein supplement.

Examples of serving sizes and approximate grams of protein are listed in the chart below.

Protein Sources ~ Serving Size ~ Grams of Protein

Food	Serving Size	Approximate Grams of Protein
Free-range chicken	3 ounces (deck of cards)	27
Grass-fed hamburger	3 ounces	22
Wild-caught fish	3 ounces	22
Lentils, soaked and then cooked	½ cup (size of child's fist)	17
Beans, soaked and then cooked	½ cup	8
Raw milk	1 cup (fist)	8
Plain yogurt	1 cup	8
Hard cheese	1 ounce (tip of thumb)	7
Free-range egg	1 large	6
Raw mixed nuts	1 ounce	5

Do You Need a Protein Supplement, Powder, or Shake?

It *is* possible to get enough protein through dietary intake. Most individuals get more than enough protein per day. However, if you are not consuming enough protein (usually if you're getting protein from only vegetable sources), it's important to look for a supplement or shake with the following components.

Avoid protein powders that have:

- more than five grams of sugar per serving
- partially hydrogenated oils as an ingredient
- artificial colors, flavors, or preservatives
- soy protein as the main source

Instead, **look for** protein powders that have:

- less than five grams of sugar per serving
- use only pure, unprocessed fats and oils, such as extra-virgin olive oil or unrefined coconut oil
- no artificial colors, flavors, or preservatives
- vegetarian or whey blend of protein

Incomplete versus Complete Protein

Think of protein (amino acids) like puzzle pieces. Some sources of protein have only a few pieces of the whole puzzle (one or more amino acid is missing). When your body has only part of the puzzle, it cannot use the protein to perform important tasks like rebuilding muscle, repairing damaged cells, or making new proteins. However, incomplete proteins are not useless. Incomplete proteins can bind together to make complete proteins. Below is a list of incomplete proteins:

- Some fruits like apples, avocados, and bananas
- Some vegetables like asparagus, cauliflower, and sweet potatoes
- Grains
- Nuts
- Legumes (peanuts and beans)

Most vegetarians get their protein from the sources listed in the previous list. When you eat the recommended daily amount of vegetables, fruits, grains, legumes, and nuts, you will consume most or all the pieces needed to complete your protein puzzle.

Complete proteins contain all the puzzle pieces necessary to make new proteins and repair your body. Complete sources include: Meat, Fish, Poultry, Eggs, Dairy

Consuming a variety is a sure way to receive other important nutrients like iron and B vitamins. Practice choosing one serving of protein for every meal and snack, and you will have a well-balanced, completed puzzle for your body's health.

Protein and Weight Management

Remember, more calories are required to break down and digest protein than to break down and absorb processed carbohydrates and sugar. Therefore, when you are consuming protein for fuel, you are burning more calories. As we learned in week 1, calories matter. Sources of protein usually have higher calories than sources of carbohydrates (i.e., vegetables), but calories from protein fill you up and leave you feeling satisfied longer. As a result, you will not be so preoccupied with your next meal or snack. Our food should nourish us, fuel us, and satisfy our hunger and our cravings. Diet food that is low in calories and nearly void of nutrients simply gives you something to chew on (or drink in a shake). Keeping your mouth busy without the necessary nutrition does not mean you are going to maintain or lose weight. Quite the opposite: chewing on empty calories usually leaves you in a state of depravity and does not lead to sustained weight loss.

Quick and Easy Protein-Packed Meal and Snack Ideas

Does ordering a pizza ever seem easier than cooking a healthy, protein-packed meal? Mealtimes are moments of opportunity. You can turn your body into a fat-burning machine with healthy, home-cooked meals, or you can allow your body to store almost everything you eat as fat with junk-food meal choices.

Use the quick-and-easy meal ideas to incorporate healthy protein into your day. Substitute any of the protein in these ideas with another variety. Look in Appendix C for even more meal ideas and recipes.

Breakfast Ideas

Avoid	Try Instead
Cereal and milk	1/2 cup 2% yogurt, 1/4 cup fruit, 1/8 cup low-sugar (10 grams or less) granola
Bagel and cream cheese	2 scrambled eggs and 1-ounce natural, hard cheese
White toast and margarine	100% whole-grain sprouted toast and 1 tablespoon butter and 1/2 cup sliced strawberries on side
Doughnut and coffee	Smoothie: 1/2 banana, 1 tablespoon almond butter, and 1 cup unsweetened coconut milk or raw whole milk
Pancakes and bacon	Homemade sourdough waffles and one whole orange

Lunch Ideas

Avoid	Try Instead
Fast-food burger	Fast-food salad with grilled chicken—dressing on the side (or skip the dressing!)
Frozen pasta meal	Frozen veggies, rice, chicken, and cheese (leftover from dinner—see below)
Sandwich with packaged meat	Salad with protein, nuts, veggies, and cheese and a slice of fresh sourdough bread on the side
Fried food or fried appetizers	Chicken skewers, beef tips, and/or salsa with celery
Canned soup high in sodium	Homemade soup with veggies and protein or canned soup with less sodium

Dinner Ideas

Avoid	Try Instead
White pasta or potatoes as the main course	Fresh or lightly steamed veggies as the main course—*get creative with new spices*
Fried food	Take a baked, steamed, or grilled approach to your traditional fried recipes
Packaged foods for most dinners	Make enough dinner to last one or two days for leftovers
Highly processed meat and veggies (think frozen dinners)	Look for meat without nitrites, nitrates, and other additives. Add wild-caught fish one to two times per week.
High-sugar desserts	2% plain yogurt with honey and fruit

Finally, the most challenging issue for most Americans: *snacks*. Snacks can make or break your food budget, your meal plan, and your scale.

Snacks

Avoid	Try Instead
Protein bars with more than 10 grams of sugar per serving	Homemade trail mix with nuts, chia seeds, no-sugar-added dried fruit, and 7 to 8 dark chocolate chips (for chocolate lovers)
Corn chips or pretzels and dip	Veggies and one serving of hummus or salsa
Candy bar	1 fruit and 1/2 cup 2% cottage cheese and 1 tablespoon almonds
Fast-food mini-meal	Lettuce wrap with protein and natural sweet chili sauce
Enriched crackers and artificial cheese dip	100% whole-grain crackers and 1 ounce of cheese

Most healthy recipes take less time to prepare than waiting for pizza delivery. As you can see, many of these meal and snack ideas call for similar ingredients. You could buy two or three pounds of chicken, a carton of plain yogurt, frozen seafood, a bag of brown rice, and a few spices, and have several different dinner ideas, all filled with healthy protein for the week (not to mention leftovers!). Add a side of steamed veggies with different spices to each entrée and you will seldom get bored with your food. Our bodies need protein to perform vital cell repair and keep us in check with a healthy weight.

If you are not already doing so, add a source of protein to each meal and snack to stay healthy and satisfied throughout the day.

How do you feel after eating protein?

What protein source (beans, chicken, fish) will you prepare this week that can last for more than one meal? Protein builds and repairs cell tissue.

How are you building and repairing your relationship with God?

Week 2, Day 6: Macronutrient – Carbohydrates

The anti-carb fad is starting to slow down a bit, but it used to be really popular. I would have people come up to me because they knew I was a nutrition expert, and they would brag, "I don't eat carbs anymore. I heard they are bad for you." This couldn't be closer to and further from the truth. There are two different classifications of carbohydrates (simple and complex), and most of them are not evil! The only kind of carbohydrate that I recommend avoiding is the processed kind. All others may be eaten in moderation. Did you know that fruits and vegetables are considered carbohydrates? It's true! And fruits and veggies are vital to your health. Let's examine this a little further, because fruits and vegetables (especially vegetables) are the best sources of carbs you can eat.

> The only kind of carbohydrate that I recommend avoiding is the processed kind.

Eat a Rainbow

The first time I was introduced to that phrase, it stuck. Did you know that the rainbow is a sign of God's covenant with Noah after the flood? In the same sense, make a covenant with your health by cherishing the *entire* rainbow of fruits and vegetables!

I encourage you to eat a rainbow as often as possible (at least every two days would be ideal). To make it even simpler, eat at least one fruit and/or vegetable with every meal and snack. Let's break that down.

Why did I specifically say to eat a rainbow? Why not eat fruits with the most antioxidants and vegetables that are highest in fiber? Or buy produce that is on sale? Those are all great places to start, but the key to produce is in the nutrients. When you eat a variety of colorful produce, you are ensuring a wide range of vitamins and minerals that your body needs and longs for. If you eat broccoli and spinach and green peppers all day, you will be well sourced in vitamin C and vitamin K, but you would be lacking vitamins A and E, which are found in orange vegetables like carrots and fruit like dried apricots. When you eat a rainbow every couple of days, you consume nourishment to fuel every cell in your body. Vitamins, minerals, and macronutrients make up the individual composition of our DNA. Illness, disease, and pain find opportunities to creep in and attack our bodies when we lack essential nutrients.

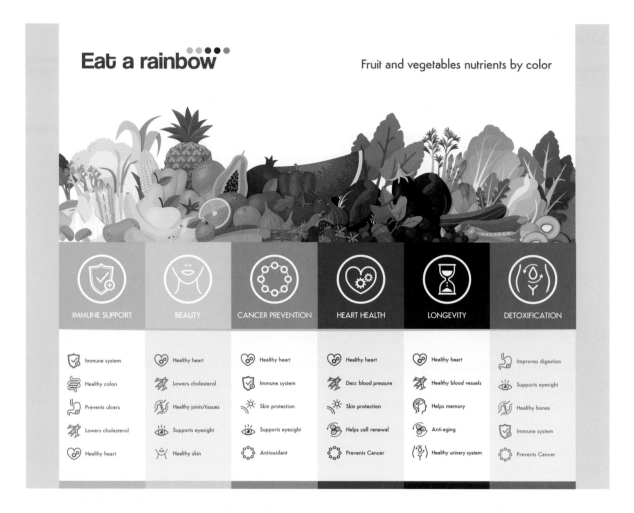

Eat a rainbow Fruit and vegetables nutrients by color

IMMUNE SUPPORT	BEAUTY	CANCER PREVENTION	HEART HEALTH	LONGEVITY	DETOXIFICATION
Immune system	Healthy heart	Healthy heart	Healthy heart	Healthy heart	Improves digestion
Healthy colon	Lowers cholesterol	Immune system	Decr. blood pressure	Healthy blood vessels	Supports eyesight
Prevents ulcers	Healthy joints/tissues	Skin protection	Skin protection	Helps memory	Healthy bones
Lowers cholesterol	Supports eyesight	Supports eyesight	Helps cell renewal	Anti-aging	Immune system
Healthy heart	Healthy skin	Antioxidant	Prevents Cancer	Healthy urinary system	Prevents Cancer

Benefits of Produce

In week 1, we examined eating for fuel *and* nourishment. Produce gives us clean fuel and ample nourishment. The benefits of eating a variety of fruits and vegetables include:

- Reduced risk of disease, diabetes, and high blood pressure. Fruits and vegetables (organic when available) help to keep you out of the doctor's office.

- Vitamins and minerals—healthy and energizing, a perfect combination

- Convenience—after you wash them, you can just grab and go! Apples in the purse, a bag of carrots in the diaper bag, or an orange in the briefcase. Produce travels well.

- Low calories—most produce is low in calories and high in satisfaction

- Antioxidants—help to remove disease-causing free radicals from your body

- Tons of fiber—natural fiber your body can break down and digest without creating a laxative effect

- Water—most are high in water content, making produce their own perfect delivery system within the fruits and vegetables to get water-soluble nutrients to the cells

- Added color and texture to your meals—presentation goes a long way. Make your meals visibly appealing and you (and your family) will be more likely to enjoy them.

Produce fills you up and is low in calories. Eat seasonal produce, usually containing nutrients you need in each season. For example, the vitamin D in fall squash helps your body store the vitamin through the winter, especially if you live in a cold climate where you may not get regular sun exposure.

Notice how you can eat certain packaged foods like ice cream and chips until the package is empty? When was the last time you finished the entire bag of lettuce or polished off three apples? One apple tastes good and is so satisfying! If you still crave certain foods after one serving, it may be time to pick a different food.

Produce is satisfying.

Weight Management

See how much more enticing the plate of vegetables and fruit is over the greasy cheeseburger on a white bun? Look at the calorie difference!

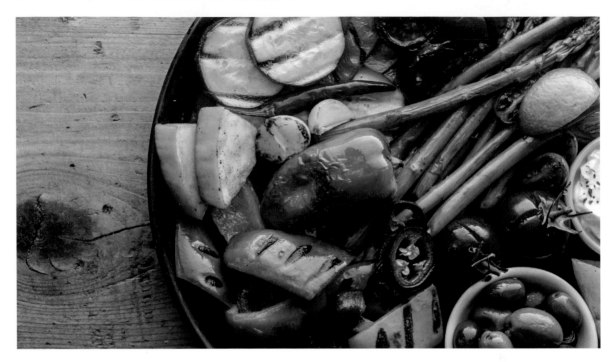

The Fruit and Veggie Plate: Approximately 300 Calories

One Cheeseburger: 1,200+ Calories

Fruits and vegetables (especially vegetables) are one of the most important food groups for losing weight and maintaining your ideal weight. Again, look at the pictures of the grill basket of veggies versus the dripping greasy burger. You can *see* the difference in nourishment. By eating a serving of vegetables at every meal, you will nourish your body with essential vitamins and minerals, fuel up with fiber for healthy digestion, and protect your cells from the leading causes of death and diseases—*with minimal calories*.

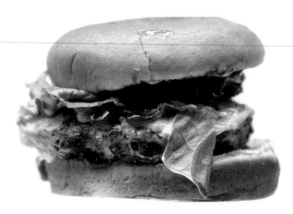

If we do nothing else but move our bodies more often, remove added sugar and processed food from our diets, and eat a variety of vegetables every day, 80 percent of the leading causes of death and disease will disappear. This proven, successful secret requires lifestyle changes, but the results ensure a healthy weight, abundant energy, and less disease.

Produce is one food group where I do not skimp. If you do not like the taste of fruits and vegetables,

> Taste is temporary; exceptional health requires a healthy lifestyle.

eat them anyway! Eventually, your palate will change. Your body craves what you eat. Eventually, your cravings subside when you refrain from eating junk food for a period of time. Sugar tastes sweet and fast food tastes awful when you haven't eaten them for a while.

Taste is temporary; exceptional health requires a healthy lifestyle.

For the health of every cell in your body, incorporate more veggies into your daily eating plan. Start with the ones you like and then add more variety to your plate over time, perhaps as they go on sale or when they are in season.

How Much Do You Need?

The government's MyPlate nutritional guide states that you need a minimum of three to five servings of fruits and vegetables per day. Yet many experts in the health and wellness industry agree that in order to meet your essential vitamin and mineral needs, you should consume a minimum of seven to nine servings of fruits and vegetables *and* take a natural multivitamin every day. I agree with the latter; more is better in this case.

Most vegetable and fruit servings are approximately the size of your fist (1/2 cup). Whole pieces of fruit, like oranges and apples, equal one serving. Leafy greens, like spinach and lettuce, equal about 1 cup per serving (uncooked).

When I encourage participants to avoid sugar and refined grains, I get the question "What can I eat? Sugar and processed foods are everywhere." You can start with vegetables and fruit! I have detailed many common veggies and fruits available, so when you feel as though your current meal plan is getting stale, you can refer to the following list and pick out something new. You have so many options of what you can eat. Grocery shopping just takes practice. Stock the right food in your fridge and pantry and be creative with new ways to plan meals. One goal that works well for me when I get sick of my same old go-tos is to eat three different colored vegetables each day and one new vegetable per month.

Grocery Shopping Woes & Encouragement from Dawn!

When you first start *Living Wellness for Growth Groups*, walking through the grocery store may feel like a new experience. Now that you're more conscious of what you are buying and putting in your body, you may feel overwhelmed with all the choices and sometimes frustrated because you can't remember what is on the Dirty Dozen list or what cancer-causing ingredient you were to stay away from. I felt very overwhelmed at first.

But don't give up or stop learning about wellness because you get overwhelmed or frustrated; your health is too important. You didn't become unhealthy overnight, so throw away the bags of shame and continue on this journey with hope! It is going to take you a while to unlearn all the unhealthy eating and exercise habits you have acquired over the years. Have patience and grace with yourself.

As you continue to open your eyes to what the food industry has done (overprocessing and adding harmful chemicals to most packaged and convenience foods), don't get mad; *just stop buying it*! I had been addicted to Diet Coke since high school; I drank it every morning until I was forty-five years old. My adrenal glands were so messed up from the artificial sweeteners that I constantly craved more sugar. Finally, I was able to kick the habit. I had headaches for weeks from the withdrawal. It was painful, but *the freedom and improved health was so worth it*. I feel better today than I have in many years!

You will be surprised when you go through the Living Wellness grocery store tour, and you discover where sugar and harmful ingredients are actually hiding. Not only is artificial sugar hiding in Diet Coke and the obvious sugar-laden candy bar but also in white bread, yogurt, cereal, coffee creamer, and bacon. Sugar, or "the white poison," causes inflammation, weight gain, obesity, and diabetes. It's time to stop neglecting your health.

Getting back to natural sugars (honey and real maple syrup), cooking real food, increasing functional exercise, and prayer are a few things that helped my health transformation. Ask God to heal *your* soul wounds. Ask God for guidance, patience, and endurance as you navigate the grocery store and try new experiences on your journey.

Living Wellness for Growth Groups is not a diet; it's a lifestyle. One change, one baby step at a time. You can do it.

Inflammation

You're going to see the word *inflammation* throughout this book. There are two kinds of inflammation in the body.

1. Acute inflammation—This is the *necessary kind* responsible for healing your body after an injury or infection.

2. Chronic inflammation—Chronic inflammation may be avoided by taking preventative measures. According to a 2007 Harvard Health publication, chronic inflammation "is the body's response to a host of modern irritations like smoking, lack of exercise, high-fat and high-calorie meals, and highly processed foods." Chronic inflammation occurs when your immune system and adrenals are overstressed. Stress is (literally) one of the leading causes of chronic inflammation. How we deal with stress greatly impacts the health of the entire body.

Chronic inflammation is linked with heart disease, diabetes, autoimmune disorders, and other chronic diseases. The more you positively change your lifestyle, *the less chronic inflammation you will have in your body*. Daily avoidance of processed foods and consuming a variety vegetables and fruit are two excellent examples of preventing chronic inflammation.

Fruit, Fruit, and More Fruit

Apple, apricot, avocado, banana, bilberry, black currant, blackberry, blueberry, cantaloupe, cherry, clementine, currant, date, eggplant, fig, gooseberry, grape, grapefruit, guava, honeydew, huckleberry, kiwi, kumquat, lemon, lime, mango, nectarine, orange, peach, pear, pineapple, plum, pomegranate, prune, raisin, raspberry, red currant, strawberry, tangerine, tomato, and watermelon. These common fruits are found at farmers' markets, grocery stores, and in your own garden!

What are different forms of fruit?

1. Fresh

2. Frozen

3. Juiced (home juiced is best)

4. Dried

5. Canned (home canned is best)

Fruit is best when it is fresh, but stocking up on a variety of forms is foresight. When you go to the grocery store, buy several servings of each of the previous sources of fruit. When you run out of fresh, you can work with your frozen, dried, or canned produce. There is such a thing as too much fruit. Remember to use the guidelines of half as much fruit per day as veggies. If you're eating four servings of veggies, aim for two different fruits per day.

What can you do with fresh or frozen fruit? Just about anything! If you use fresh fruit in the smoothie recipes below, throw in a couple of ice cubes or plain yogurt to thicken.

Delicious and Nutritious Fruit Smoothie Recipes

Strawberry Banana Smoothie

Serves 1

1/2 cup fresh or frozen strawberries: 39 calories
1 frozen banana: 110 calories
1 cup unsweetened almond or coconut milk: 45 calories
1 tablespoon fresh ground flax seeds*: 55 calories
Total calories: 249

Blueberry Banana Smoothie

Serves 1

1/4 cup fresh or frozen blueberries: 20 calories
1 fresh or frozen banana: 110 calories
1 cup unsweetened almond or coconut milk: 45 calories
1 tablespoon real maple syrup: 50 calories (optional)
Total calories: 225

Pineapple Mango Smoothie with Granola

Serves 1

1/2 cup fresh or frozen pineapple mango strawberry fruit blend 100% fruit, no sugar added: 47 calories
1 cup unsweetened almond or coconut milk: 45 calories
2 tablespoons low-sugar granola: 70 calories
1 tablespoon chia seeds*: 65 calories
Total calories: 227

*Flax and chia seeds are excellent sources of protein and healthy fats and they usually blend well in smoothies.

These recipes are delicious for breakfast or a midmorning snack (or even dessert!). You can substitute any fresh or frozen fruits for your favorite kinds. You can also substitute the almond or coconut milk for regular milk. Nondairy milk offers calcium without added side effects often found in cow milk, and avoiding dairy may be more beneficial for individuals with asthma and certain respiratory and skin conditions.

Dried or dehydrated fruits are great for salads, yogurt embellishments, homemade trail mixes, rice pilafs, and homemade baked goods (among others). Dried cranberries and cherries are great for all of the above ideas. Dried blueberries are great in granola or baked goods. When you add your own mineral salt, dried bananas and plantains are good for salty snacking, and dried tropical fruit makes for a great dessert alone or with yogurt. Dried fruits may often contain large amounts of added sugar, so look for brands without any added sugar (or processed oil, for that matter).

Canned fruit is an acceptable source when you are out of fresh or frozen fruit. Canned fruit is also nice to have on hand if you cannot get to the grocery store, or if your budget does not allow you to always buy fresh. Also, choose fruit that is canned with 100 percent fruit juice rather than heavy or lite syrup, or even artificial sugar, such as Splenda®. The price is usually the same, but the health benefits of fruit are lessened when drenched in sticky, sugary corn syrup. Canned fruit is good on its own or paired with cottage cheese, yogurt, or salad. Children and mature adults sometimes prefer canned fruit because it is much softer and easier to eat. However, choose canned produce sparingly to avoid excess aluminum and/or plastic ingestion. *Do not rely on canned goods as your main source of produce.*

Veggies, Veggies, and More Veggies

Below is a long list of vegetables and plants that are available at most grocery stores. Take this list to the store and purchase one new vegetable each month. Learn how to prepare and cook that veggie in multiple different ways or make the same recipe a few times. Think of the veggie repertoire you will have after a year! **Also, make it a goal to eat at least one veggie daily at every meal and snack!**

Artichoke, arugula, asparagus, bamboo, beans, beet, bok choy, broccoli, Brussels sprouts, cabbage, capers, carrot, celery, chard, collards, corn, cucumber, eggplant, endive, fennel, garbanzo, garlic, ginger, ginseng, horseradish, jicama, jojoba, kale, leek, lentils, lettuce, melon, mushroom, okra, onion, paprika, parsley, parsnip, peas, pepper, pimiento, potato, pumpkin, radicchio, radish, rhubarb, romaine lettuce, rutabaga, saffron, sea kale, shallot, soybeans, spinach, squash, sweet potato, and yams.

Which vegetables will you try first for your "one new vegetable per month" routine?

_____

_____

_____

_____

What are different forms of vegetables?

1. Fresh
2. Frozen
3. Juiced (home juiced is best)
4. Dried
5. Canned (home canned is best)

Fresh is always best, but variety is also wise! Stock up on fresh, frozen, dried, and canned to provide texture, taste, and—most importantly—nutrients into every meal and snack.

What do you do with your favorite vegetables?

I keep a variety of frozen veggies on hand for the times I run out of fresh. Sometimes I toss whatever frozen veggies I have in my wok and make a stir-fry surprise! Avoid buying frozen vegetables with added ingredients. The ingredient label should just say what the vegetable is, nothing more.

There are days when I get tired of preparing and eating vegetables. I know that eating veggies is vital to staying healthy and energized, so when I just don't feel like eating one more bite of carrot, I get out my juicer. I started juicing a few years ago, and the results have been so encouraging. My favorite combinations include carrots, cucumbers, beets, spinach, and ginger (not a vegetable, but ginger adds so much flavor and healthful benefits). Get creative! You can juice almost anything you can think of. Also, juicing is a fabulous way to get your kids to try new foods. After months of drinking beet juice, both my children now enjoy roasted beets! My son loves beet, carrot, and apple juice, especially when he gets to help make it! Juicing is also a way to use up mushy (but not rotten) vegetables and fruits. Apples, celery, carrots, spinach, chard, oranges, and grapefruits are just a few fruits and veggies I have managed to save with the juicer. Not many people enjoy eating a mushy orange, but everyone enjoys fresh orange juice!

Most of the fiber is discarded during the juicing process, unless you use the pulp for soup, muffins, or stir-fry, so be sure that juicing is not your main source of vegetable consumption. Juicing is a great treat once in a while. Also, if you're buying juice rather than making it yourself, look for juice with no added sugar, preservatives, or colors.

Dried veggies are great for snacking. Dehydrated green beans and snap peas are popular for their flavor, texture, and healthy qualities. Dried beans are a wonderful addition to soups, salads, wraps, and a stir-fry (you will need to first soak and cook dried beans).

Canned vegetables can be good to throw into a stir-fry when you are low on fresh veggies, and they are also great on a salad; try canned artichoke hearts on your favorite salad or homemade pizza for a boost of protein (yes, protein!), vitamin C, vitamin K, folate (good for the brain), magnesium, omegas, and fiber—wow! All this from a canned veggie (or fresh if you prepare artichoke hearts)! These nutrients fuel your body, protect your brain, and keep your body free from disease and malnourishment.

The colorful roasted root vegetable salad below is delicious alongside broiled steaks or oven-baked ribs. Use any variety of sweet potato you like, including the ones sometimes labeled "garnet yams," which have a bright orange color and moist, sweet flesh.

Salad Recipe

Roasted Sweet Potato Salad with Pecans and Green Onions

Original recipe modified from Williams-Sonoma Salad of the Day

Serves 4-6

3 pounds (1.5 kilograms) sweet potatoes
2 tablespoons virgin olive oil
Mineral salt and pre-ground pepper
1/2 cup pecans
1/3 cup fresh lime juice
3 tablespoons real maple syrup
1/2 cup minced green onions, including tender green parts
3-4 leaves kale, stemmed and leaves torn

Preheat the oven to 400 degrees Fahrenheit. Peel the sweet potatoes and cut them into 1-inch chunks. Put them in a large baking pan, drizzle with 1 1/2 tablespoons of the oil, sprinkle with 1/2 teaspoon salt, and mix to coat. Spread the sweet potatoes in a single layer and roast, stirring occasionally until tender when pierced with a knife, 25-30 minutes.

Meanwhile, in a dry frying pan, toast the pecans over medium-low heat, stirring until fragrant and starting to brown, about 5 minutes. Slide onto a plate to cool.

In a large bowl, mix the lime juice, maple syrup, and remaining 1/2 tablespoon oil. Add the hot roasted sweet potatoes to the lime juice mixture along with the pecans, green onions, and torn kale. Mix well and season with pepper and additional salt. Serve at once or let cool to room temperature and mix again before serving.

The stir-fry recipe below is wonderful in mid-summer when your garden eggplant is ready to harvest. Feel free to swap out any veggies for the ones you have on hand.

Stir-fry is a great way to use up those "back-of-fridge veggies" or try some new varieties. This recipe is especially tasty and colorful!

Stir-Fry Recipe

Original recipe modified from Williams-Sonoma

Serves 4

2 tablespoons unrefined coconut oil
1 red bell pepper, cored, seeded, and julienned
1 yellow bell pepper, cored, seeded, and julienned
1/2 cup red onion, thinly sliced
1 cup yellow squash, half-moon sliced
1 cup small broccoli florets
1 baby eggplant, cut into chunks
8 ounces chicken or steak, cut into large chunks
1 clove garlic, minced
1/2 cup teriyaki sauce (check the label: no more than 2 grams sugar per serving)
2 cups sliced bok choy
1 cup fresh mung bean sprouts
1/4 teaspoon freshly ground black pepper
1/4 teaspoon mineral salt
1/2 cup snow peas
2 tablespoons sesame oil

Start by preparing and cutting all the vegetables and measuring your ingredients so that they are ready to go. Once you begin stir-frying, the next steps go quickly.

In a wok or large skillet, heat coconut oil over high heat until almost smoking. Add the peppers and onion while stirring constantly. Add successively the squash, broccoli, eggplant, chicken or steak, garlic, and teriyaki sauce. Cook, stirring constantly for 2 minutes. Add the bok choy, sprouts, pepper, and salt, and cook, stirring, until crisp-tender, about 2 minutes more.

Stir in snow peas and sesame oil and remove from heat. Serve immediately.

The cooking time for this tasty dish is only ten minutes! There is a little prep, but it's worth it—and it's still quicker than ordering takeout.

Grilled Fish and Summer Squash

Serves 4

2 teaspoons Dijon mustard
Lemon zest, grated from 1 lemon
2 tablespoons fresh lemon juice
1/3 cup (plus more as needed) virgin or extra-virgin olive oil
1 small serrano chili, seeded and minced
1 teaspoon minced fresh marjoram
1 teaspoon minced fresh basil
Coarse mineral salt and fresh ground pepper
1 pound of your favorite fish, cut in chunks (mahimahi or tuna steak works well for skewers)
8 summer squash, cut lengthwise into 3 pieces each

Soak bamboo skewers in water and cover for 30 minutes. Prepare a charcoal or gas grill for direct- heat cooking over medium-high heat.

Add the mustard to a small bowl and stir in lemon zest and juice, mixing well. Gradually whisk in 1/3 cup olive oil. Mix in the chili and herbs. Season the sauce to taste with salt and pepper.

Skewer the fish. Arrange the squash on the grill, cover, and cook until tender and lightly charred, about 5 minutes per side. Transfer to a plate. Place the fish skewers on the grill and cook, uncovered, until just cooked through, about 4 minutes per side. Remove the fish from the skewers and cut the squash crosswise. Transfer the fish and squash to a medium bowl and toss with the lemon-herb sauce. Season to taste with salt and pepper and serve immediately.

Quick tips: Vary the recipe by using red bell peppers in place of summer squash or scallops instead of fish. Chicken breasts are also good with these seasonings. To save time, make the dressing one day ahead and refrigerate. Bring it to room temperature before using.

Should You Go Organic?

Yes! When choosing produce, always look for certified organic products. Most nonorganic produce carries potential chemicals like pesticides, herbicides, and preservatives that are harmful to your thyroid and metabolism. These chemicals are also linked to chronic inflammation, which is a contributing factor to most leading causes of death and disease. If 100 percent organic produce is not in the budget, refer to the EWG Guide in Appendix D to look up the Dirty Dozen and Clean Fifteen produce list.

How Many Vegetable Servings Do You Need Per Day?

Remember, you need at least three to five servings of veggies per day (five to seven servings of produce total).

Eating Clean—Is It More Expensive?

Most fruits and veggies are low in calories and high in nourishment. Produce also supplies heart-healthy fiber, which is responsible for absorbing toxins and sweeping them out of our body.

I often hear that eating healthily is too expensive. This is simply not true. Initially, we may take more time to learn how to grocery shop and cook with healthy ingredients, but eating clean, whole foods is not more expensive in the long run. How much money do we spend on empty-calorie foods—chips, ice cream, soda, candy bars—in the checkout lane? One bag of chips can cost more than three dollars for just seven ounces, versus similar spending on a half dozen organic peaches in season. Studies have proven that replacing junk food with whole food provides cost savings now and long term; consuming healthy food allows us to be more productive at home and work, sleep better, have fewer mental health problems, and manage our ideal weight.

Being healthier reduces medical costs. Consuming quality produce is an investment in your health.

The cost savings from eating clean are tangible. They are not just produce-in-the-sky suggestions that may or may not happen with improved health. When you fuel and nourish your body with the right foods and the right amounts, you will be healthier. You will feel better. You will save money, short term and long term.

Let's add up all the money we will save by consistently eating clean.

- How much will you save by cutting down on junk food, fast food, and eating out?
- How much will you save by not missing work due to your (or your child's) illness?
- How much will you save by not purchasing fiber supplements, weight loss pills, or diet programs?
- How much will you save by avoiding that sleep study or drugs to help you sleep (or help you snore less)?
- How much will you save by avoiding drugs to keep you awake? Gourmet coffee is expensive.
- How much will you save by reducing the need for mental health care, for issues such as anxiety and depression?
- How much will you save when you no longer need to buy larger clothes?
- How much will you save when you reduce visits to the doctor's office because of preventable illness or disease?

Estimate how much money you could save by eating clean and exercising consistently:

$ _____

I facilitated a grocery store tour not long ago. As we began the tour, one gentleman was commenting about his love affair with sugar, coffee, and wine. As we continued, he complained about the cost of healthy food. He said he just wasn't convinced that eating healthily was worth it to him at this stage in his life. As we were walking out of the grocery store, he stopped and said, "I have to go back. I forgot to get my antacids." It struck me that this man wouldn't think twice about buying drugs to treat the symptoms of acid reflux, yet a few simple nutritional changes would cure the acid reflux altogether. Eating healthier would not only prevent the painful acid reflux, but it would also give him more energy and a more vibrant life.

I occasionally find myself looking for the quick fix in a situation. Usually, however, the quick fix is simply putting a Band-Aid on a broken arm; it doesn't solve the root of the problem. Cutting corners to save costs may seem thrifty in the short term, but the fuel you put in your body becomes you. Consistently nourishing your body will save money in the long run, and you'll reap all the positive benefits of eating healthily right now—think of it as an immediate investment into your abundant life!

> Usually, however, the quick fix is simply putting a Band-Aid on a broken arm; it doesn't solve the root of the problem.

Week 2, Day 7: Recap & Reflect

- Focus on what you're doing well and keep doing it! Celebrate small successes.

- Your metabolism is complex, but you have the ability to either make it work for you or against you. Improve your metabolism by eating breakfast and then small, consistent meals throughout the day, drinking plenty of water, consistently strength training your muscles, and keeping your plate filled with vegetables, protein, healthy fat, and small amounts of fermented foods and fruit. Avoid processed foods as much as possible.

- Ingredients to avoid include preservatives, flavor enhancers and artificial sweeteners, enriched grains, and artificial colors and flavors. You are what you eat! Fill your body with nourishing fuel, not toxic waste.

- Digestion governs the inner workings of your body. You can improve digestion and absorption by chewing your food thoroughly, slowing down, and relaxing during and after your meals as much as possible.

- Protein is the vital building block for all cells. Protein also repairs cell damage. Consume a healthy, complete protein at each meal and snack. Good sources of protein include meat, fish, beans, nuts, seeds, poultry, eggs, and (some) dairy. Aim for three to five servings per day.

- Drink at least half of your ideal body weight in ounces of filtered water daily in order to hydrate your brain and muscles, transport nutrients to your cells, aid in your digestion, and flush your liver and kidneys.

- Carbohydrates are not evil. They are an essential macronutrient. Fruits and vegetables, especially vegetables, are your best sources of healthy, low-calorie carbs. Aim for a minimum of five to seven servings of vegetables and fruits per day, twice as many vegetables as fruits. Eat a variety of colors (think about the rainbow) to get a plethora of vitamins and minerals.

- Cutting corners to save costs may seem thrifty in the short term, but the fuel you put into your body becomes you. Consistently nourishing your body will save money in the long run, and you'll reap all the positive benefits of eating healthily right now—think of it as an immediate investment into your abundant life!

How did your action steps impact your health goal this week?

_____

_____

_____

_____

As you're gaining more knowledge about your body, did any new health goals come to mind? If so, go back to week 1, day 7 and use the provided space to write them out.

What was challenging this week?

_____

_____

_____

What did you do well?

_____

_____

_____

Knowledge is empowering. Use it wisely!

Reflection Notes:

_____

_____

_____

_____

_____

_____

_____

_____

_____

_____

_____

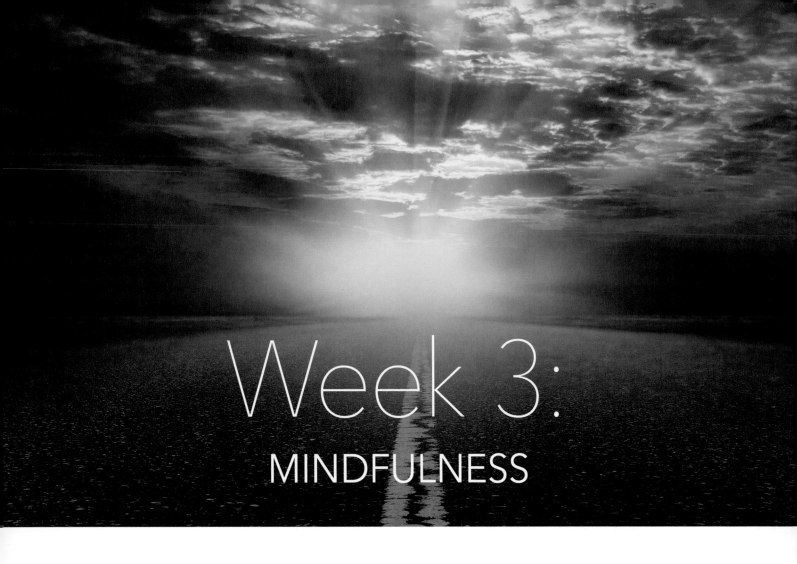

Week 3:
MINDFULNESS

This week, we will learn how to practice mindful eating and examine mindfulness in several areas of our health and habits. Being mindful means to slow down and think about what you're doing and why you're doing it. You can practice mindfulness in any and all areas of your life! This week, we will focus on mindful eating.

**Our awareness of our harmful habits
is the first step to changing them.**

Mindful Eating

I was running around the house, anxious about a deadline, when my sister (who is an occupational therapist) called. I told her I was about to eat the entire kitchen (which is my instinct when I'm anxious). She prayed with me and then told me to get an orange. I said, "What does an orange have to do with my anxiety?"

She said, "Trust me."

So I grabbed an orange, and over the phone, she talked me through the following exercise.

Unbeknownst to her, this changed my entire way of eating. My sister learned the following technique from a psychologist as a calming and focusing exercise, but as a nutrition expert, I had other ideas about its application.

The benefits of mindful eating include learning when to start and stop eating, learning to better manage emotional eating, practicing being present, improving digestion and absorption of your food, and increasing your awareness of how you feel after you eat. If you are part of a Living Wellness Growth Group, you will do mindful eating together. However, you are welcome and encouraged to practice on your own as well!

This exercise works best with an organic citrus fruit, such as an orange or grapefruit, but be encouraged to practice mindful eating at *every meal and snack*. If you are allergic to citrus fruits, practice with an apple, pear, or a half-cup of strawberries instead (skip the peeling).

Practice Mindful Eating with Me

Step 1: Hold the fruit in your hands. Carefully take in the sight. Notice the color, shape, and texture. Focus only on the fruit. Take a deep breath.

Step 2: Peel the fruit (if applicable). Notice the smell, the color change, and the texture. Continue breathing deeply and relax your shoulders.

Step 3: Put one small piece of the fruit in your mouth. Notice the taste, the smell, and the texture. Chew slowly. Breathe deeply.

Step 4: Continue eating the rest of the fruit, slowly, taking in all the senses as you eat.

Step 5: Notice how you feel after you have eaten the fruit. Do you feel satisfied? Do you feel good?

Step 6: Once you're finished eating, let go of thoughts about food. The inability to release thoughts about food is at the root of our most challenging eating habits. Moving away from thoughts about food gives us the freedom to direct mental and emotional energy toward God. Be glad for the experience, and be satisfied with your choice of fruit and the amount. Let your mind move away from food and on to giving thanks.

Step 7: Give thanks. Thank God and ask him to nourish your body with the fruit.

Practice mindful eating daily.

After practicing mindful eating, what are your thoughts?

_____

_____

_____

How do you feel after practicing the exercise? How do you feel thirty minutes later?

_____

_____

Do you feel satisfied or do you want more food?

_____

How will practicing mindful eating transform your health and your relationship with food?

_____

_____

When will you practice mindful eating each day of this week?

_____

_____

We would be wise to practice mindfulness in all areas of our lives. How can you practice mindfulness to improve your relationship with God?

_____

_____

God desires us to enjoy our food with great pleasure—not just the taste but the experience. Why else did he give us a nose, taste buds, and endorphins? Next time you eat, use all your senses and enjoy the experience! Then, remember to rest while you digest.

Week 3 Action Steps

Number one health goal: _____ *Goal Accomplished!* ☐

Accountability

Record your **strength** workouts in the *Living Wellness Journal*;

weekly goal:_____ _____ (number of days) (minutes per day) ☐

    Partner's goal: _____ _____ (number of days) (minutes per day)

Record your **cardio** workouts in the *Living Wellness Journal*;

weekly goal:_____ _____ (number of days) (minutes per day) ☐

    Partner's goal: _____ _____ (number of days) (minutes per day)

What is your **nutrition** goal this week (remember the SMART goals)? _____ ☐

    Partner's nutrition goal: _____ ☐

Record your **food/beverage** intake in *Living Wellness Journal* or app ☐

Check in with your partner daily. ☐ ☐ ☐ ☐ ☐ ☐

Knowledge

Fill out all questions in this book *prior* to the next meeting. ☐

Mindfulness

Practice mindful eating daily. ☐ ☐ ☐ ☐ ☐ ☐

Inspiration

Make a habit out of giving thanks to God before or after eating. ☐ ☐ ☐ ☐ ☐ ☐

Motivation

Why do you want to be free from the cycle of sugar addiction? What or who could you spend

that extra energy on? _____

Living Wellness Week 3 Exercises

Add these two exercises to your existing strength training routine.

Dumbbell Squat (dumbbells optional)

Stand with your feet hip-width apart. Keeping the weight even on the bottoms of your feet, inhale as you bend your knees and stick your butt back, like you're going to sit on a chair. Keep your chest and head up. Exhale as you squeeze your butt muscles and stand up. Keep your core tight by pulling your midsection in.

For Option II, add an upright row as you stand up from your squat. Keep your wrists straight and elbows in line with your shoulders.

Perform 16 to 20 reps. Repeat as time permits.

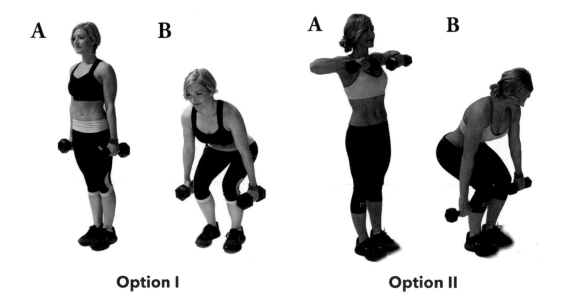

Option I   **Option II**

Dumbbell Bent-Over Row

With a neutral spine, hinge forward until your back is at about a 45-degree angle. Keep your knees slightly bent the whole time. Draw your core in tightly and inhale as you drop your hands directly below your shoulders. Exhale as you pull your elbows up to be parallel with your shoulders.

For Option II, start in a split stance (lunge position) and alternate arms rather than pulling both up at the same time.

Perform 16 to 20 reps or for the single-arm rows, 8 to 10 reps on each arm/leg. Repeat as time permits. Practice these exercises every other day. Stretch your muscles after your workout.

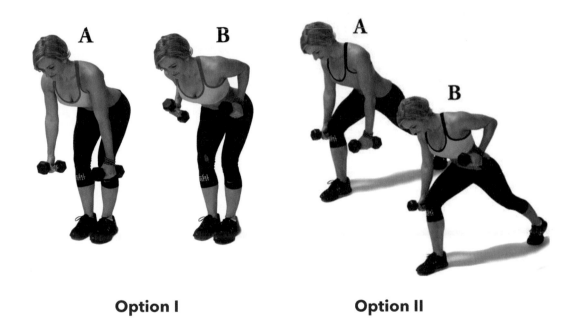

Option I　　　　　**Option II**

Looking Ahead

This week we will look at sugar (and food) addictions and their consequences, how to reduce sugar cravings, and how to replace our sugar foods with delicious, life-giving foods. This is an important week!

Week 3, Day 2: Are You Addicted to Sugar?

I was amazed to learn that there is not one single function within my body that requires added *sugar. Eat carrots, it will help your eyesight; eat spinach, it will boost your iron. Eat sugar and you will wreck everything you've tried so hard to fix.*

—Tracy S., trusted friend and mentor

We are an over-sugared nation. Most people are addicted to sugar and *all the foods that turn to sugar quickly in our bodies* (we'll tackle those in day 4). Sugar is killing us, slowly and painfully. There is added sugar in almost every processed and packaged food. There is added sugar in almost every sports drink and alcoholic drink, and now there is talk of adding sugar to milk! Milk has natural sugar (lactose), but it shouldn't be listed on the ingredient label! If there is more than just "milk" (and sometimes Vitamin D3) listed on the ingredient label, choose a different brand! For most individuals, consuming sugar from natural sources, such as fruit, vegetables, dairy, real honey, and maple syrup, produces no negative effects; it is the overwhelming amount of sugar that has been *added to our foods* that is getting us all addicted.

Effects of Sugar on the Brain

Sugar affects the same "feel-good" brain hormones as street drugs. A participant in one of my Living Wellness Growth Groups admitted once, "I could walk away from the heroin. I can't walk away from food. I need it, and I'm addicted."

The scientific community is waking up to that fact that sugar and processed carbs activate the same reward centers in our brains as addictive drugs. When you *overload* on sugary foods, they alter your appetite control center. In lab studies, rats that binged on sugar had brain changes like those addicted to drugs.

In human testing, just *seeing* pictures of milkshakes *triggered brain effects like those seen in drug addicts*.

Why Are We Addicted?

Bad habits and addictions are complicated. For food, the response is both a:

- Physical addiction
  - Hormones
  - Brain
  - Tongue
- Psychological addiction
  - Habitual
  - Emotional
  - Social

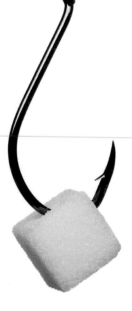

Are *you* addicted to sugar, carbs, alcohol, or food? I know I have struggled with a lifetime sugar addiction. Take this quiz to examine your relationship with sugar (or food or even alcohol) addiction.

Addiction Survey

Addictions are hard to define; there are physical and psychological addictions. Proving something is an addiction is a bit difficult, but the test below is an assessment that may work for any addiction, including sugar. Be honest in your answers.

- **Have you ever used sugar/carbs/food/alcohol as a reward for something?** Was sugar the treat you gave yourself after you completed a task or a job well done? Yes/No

- **Have you ever used sugar/carbs/food/alcohol to change your mood**, like when you felt sad, tired, or when you needed a lift? Yes/No

- **Have you ever eaten sugar/carbs/food/alcohol even when you weren't hungry?** You just finished a meal and are very full, but still you order dessert or go to the fridge and pull out the ice cream. Yes/No

- **Have you ever tried to stop eating sugar/carbs/food/alcohol and couldn't?** You tried a diet like Atkins or South Beach but felt endlessly drawn by sugar and foods that act like sugar and couldn't stick to the diet. Yes/No

- **Have you ever taken a small bite of something sweet and felt compelled to finish the whole thing?** You thought you were just going to have a bite of something, but then you ate the whole thing. Processed foods count here too: Have you ever started to eat a few potato or corn chips and finished the whole bag? Yes/No

- **Have you ever quit eating sugar/carbs/food/alcohol for a time and when you started eating it again, couldn't stop bingeing?** When you took sugar out of your diet and then returned to it, did you binge on sugar and sugary foods? Yes/No

If you answered yes to one or two of these questions, then you probably have a sugar problem. If you answered yes to two or more of these questions, then you are guaranteed to be addicted to sugar/carbs/or food.

What are your thoughts about this survey?

_____

_____

_____

The signs of addiction are typically:

- Using the addiction for a reward
- Consuming the substance to change your mood
- Feeling compelled to consume the addiction even though you don't need it
- Bingeing, especially when the addicted substance is removed for a while

Before you dismiss sugar addiction as a funny thing we all have, you need to realize that any food or beverage addiction ultimately means harm to your body; excess sugar consumption is associated with increased weight and obesity, diabetes, heart disease, and potentially many other diseases.

If you have known or you are just realizing that you are addicted to sugar, carbs, food, or anything, give it to God! Admit you are powerless to change on your own. Ask God to give you the desire to be set free and the strength to make small daily changes. I pray with you that you will be intrinsically motivated to change your eating habits. Lysa Terkeurst, author of *Made to Crave: Satisfying Your Deepest Desire with God, Not Food*, states that *we crave what we eat*! When we reduce the consumption of sugar-filled and processed foods, we begin to crave them less! Reduced cravings are worth the fight. When we eliminate them altogether, we will see the transformation in every area of our health.

Addressing your sugar addiction can be challenging, but if you have the desire, you can change with proper support, education, and help. Ask God right now (if you are ready) to plant the seed of *freedom* in your heart. Then continue learning about your body and prepare yourself to take action!

Start Reducing Sugar Cravings Today:

1. Write down your goals. Are you planning on cutting your sugar consumption in half? How often will you go out to eat? How often will you have desserts? Write down your goals and then share them with trusted friends and family to help you stay on track. Track your progress in the *Living Wellness Journal* or nutrition app.

2. Out of sight, out of mind: get the junk food out of the house! If you were an alcoholic, you would get rid of all the alcohol in your house. The same is true with addictive junk food: out of sight, *out of arm's reach*, out of mind.

3. Keep plenty of low-sugar fruits, fresh and/or frozen strawberries, blackberries, raspberries, and green apples in the house to help satisfy sugar cravings.

4. Look for treats that are sweetened naturally with fruit, honey, or real maple syrup. For example, LÄRABAR is a company that makes brownie bites sweetened with dates rather than table sugar. If you have other members in your household that bring in junk food, ask them to put their food in a high cupboard—away from your eyesight and reach.

5. Try glutamine! Glutamine is a supplement that has been proven to reduce sugar and alcohol cravings. Follow instructions on the label.

6. Retrain your habits. Instead of having dessert after each meal, take a walk, play a game, or share a funny memory from the day.

7. Before you reach for your next meal or snack, ask yourself, *will this food or beverage nourish my body or simply provide fuel?*

If you practice making changes and the cravings or addictions still have a grip on you, take heart. Just because this is your struggle now, does not mean this is how you will always be. Keep practicing, and submit your challenges to God. Admit you are powerless to change on your own and ask for a change of heart (and cravings!) and then continue nourishing your body to the best of your ability. Remember, you crave what you eat: *focus more on filling your body with healthy, nourishing foods*, rather than focusing so hard on what you're *trying to avoid*. Use the recipe below for an easy, delicious, and healthy treat—containing zero grams of processed sugar!

Sea Salt Cocoa-Covered Almonds
—Ashley's Favorite Dessert Recipe (Serves 1)

Ingredients
1 tablespoon almond butter
1 teaspoon raw honey (locally sourced honey is best)
1 tablespoon raw cocoa powder
1 tablespoon unrefined coconut oil
1/4 teaspoon sea salt or mineral salt (use only a small pinch)
1/8 cup raw almonds or pecans

Directions
In a small saucepan, heat almond butter and coconut oil on low until melted. Remove from heat. Add honey, cocoa powder, and salt, mixing well. Sprinkle the nuts in the mixture and enjoy! You can eat this treat with a spoon or dip in your favorite fruit. If you want to make the mixture into a homemade protein and fiber bar, scoop the mixture onto wax paper and let it cool in the fridge.
Calories: 270

What new habits will you create to support your healthy lifestyle (one that manages addiction)?

_____

_____

_____

What have you learned about yourself thus far in your journey?

_____

_____

_____

_____

_____

Use this space to write a prayer to God. Give him your struggles and addictions. Ask God to take them from you. Then allow the Holy Spirit to lead you and your choices with food.

_____

_____

_____

_____

_____

_____

_____

_____

_____

_____

_____

_____

_____

_____

_____

_____

_____

Week 3, Day 3: Processed Carbs – The Nonfood That's Keeping You Addicted

John 5:6: "When Jesus saw him lying there and learned that he had been in this condition for a long time, he asked him, *'Do you want to get well*?'" [Italics mine]

One day, several years ago, one of my clients quit eating foods with added sugar in hopes of getting control of crazy food cravings. The client had some success. She mentioned the cravings did go down some and that she lost weight but that some foods still triggered massive sugar cravings and the weight loss plateaued at a certain point.

I encouraged her to keep a food journal to help determine what triggered the cravings. It didn't take long before my client realized that every time she binged on foods like pizza, cereal, bagels, pasta, and crackers, the cravings would come back with a vengeance and the number on her scale hit a standstill. She was confused because the foods listed didn't necessarily have added sugar in them. But all those foods have something in common: they are highly processed carbohydrates.

Processed carbohydrates often confuse people when it comes to sugar addiction because when you look at the ingredient label of a bag of pasta, there is usually no sugar listed. However, you may see an ingredient called "enriched flour."

Processed carbs and enriched grains, such as white bread, most boxed crackers, muffins, cereal, and white pasta, *turn to sugar quickly in our bodies*, creating the same spike-crash hormone response as plain old table sugar. And processed carbs are high in calories, low in protein, low in fiber, and not satisfying.

Imagine eating a fast-food hamburger and instead of the bun, you ate bun-shaped sugar cubes! Or instead of a warm bagel with cream cheese, you ate a bagel-shaped sugar cube with cream cheese. Or perhaps, the worst is imagining your plate full of pasta noodles turning into—you guessed it, a plate full of sugar cubes drizzled with tomato paste. *Ugh!* When we eat processed—or *enriched*—grains, we might as well be eating sugar cubes, void of most digestible and absorbable nutrition.

We often crave sugar after eating processed carbs because of the quick energy we feel, but that rush does not last long.

Similar to sugar, overconsuming processed carbs results in a roller coaster of a day—a roller coaster of blood sugar and energy level swings, depression, anxiety, hormone imbalance, body aches, brain fog, obesity, and disease.

> Removing processed carbs from your diet is the secret weapon to reducing sugar cravings once and for all.

Frozen waffle or bagel for breakfast, spike and crash; fat-free "diet" crackers for a snack, spike and crash; white flour sandwich and chips with lunch, spike and crash. Removing processed carbs from your diet is the secret weapon to reducing sugar cravings once and for all.

My husband and I went out to eat a while back and he was deciding between the nachos and salmon salad. He had a long day at work and was tired, thus, giving in to the nachos. After dinner he looked at me with that familiar regretful look on his face and said, *I should have had the salmon*.

I used to fight the same battle—*give in to my taste buds or eat something nourishing? Should not or should?* Thankfully, God showed me that the consequences weren't worth giving in to my temporary cravings. It's not out of some religious law or fear that I eat healthy. I eat healthy because I have the freedom to do so, and I desire to honor God with my choices. *Being made well along the way is an absolutely delightful result.*

> I eat healthy because I have the freedom to do so, and I desire to honor God with my choices. Being made well along the way is an absolutely delightful result.

In order to *be made well*, to heal our bodies from the damage of too much sugar, and begin to break free from the chains of sugar cravings, we must do some hard work and change habits, starting by being mindful of everything we put in our mouths.

In talking through why he makes the choices he does, my husband is making better choices at restaurants and at home more often than not. This didn't happen overnight. We have been married ten years. But he is now healthier because he *made the decision* that he wanted to be healthier. Then he started making decisions based off that choice. My husband is thirty-five pounds lighter today than he was two years ago. He really wanted to break free from the cycle of sugar addiction, and he did. I'm so proud of him and the example he is setting for our children. Be encouraged, you can change too.

Be honest here. Do you really *want to* change? Do you want to be free from food addictions? Do you want to be healed from issues that are causing you to make consistently poor choices?

What will your life look like once these changes occur?

_____

_____

_____

What changes will you make in order to move toward a life of freedom with your health?

_____

_____

Week 3, Day 4: Consequences of Sugar Addiction

Hopefully by now you realize that food addictions are real and that sugar and processed carb addictions are as strong as heroin! Let's examine the side effects of eating for reasons other than nourishment.

Harmful (and expensive) effects of consuming too much sugar:

- Heart disease
- Obesity
- Diabetes
- Chronic diseases
- High blood pressure
- Chronic inflammation
- Increased triglycerides
- Tooth decay

The harmful effects of overconsumption or addiction go way beyond the obvious:

- Shame
- Low self-esteem
- Unhealthy body image
- Family turmoil because of mood swings

Heart Disease

If you think I'm blowing the issue of sugar and processed food addiction out of proportion, take a look at some heart disease stats from the Centers for Disease Control and Prevention website:

- About **611,000 people** die of heart disease in the United States every year— that's **1 in every 4 deaths**.
- Heart disease is the leading cause of death for both men and women. **More than half** of the deaths due to heart disease in 2009 were in men.
- Coronary heart disease is the most common type of heart disease, killing more than **370,000 people** annually.
- Every year, about **735,000 Americans** have a heart attack. Of these, 525,000 are a first heart attack, and **210,000 happen in people who have already had a heart attack.**
- Coronary heart disease alone costs the United States **$108.9 billion** each year. This total includes the cost of health care services, medications, and lost productivity.

There's no need to focus on the aspects of your health that you can't change, such as your family history or age. Instead, step into the reality of your situation, make a plan, and focus on the controllable factors of your health.

Weight Gain

Sugary cereal or a muffin for breakfast, spike and crash; packaged snack cake or candy for a treat, spike and crash; cookie and soda with lunch, spike and crash; dessert after dinner, you guessed it, spike and crash. Sounds like our spike-crash day from eating processed carbs, doesn't it? Continuing this pattern results in feeling so hungry by the end of the day that you eat every available packaged food in the pantry. If you took the time to add up all the empty calories from the day, you would most likely be appalled.

Eating too many high-calorie, low-satiety foods leads to weight gain—you want more because the foods and beverages you are consuming lack essential nutrients and keep your body in want! Guess what? If you eat like that on a regular basis, you are teaching your body to *crave* junk food, void of anything truly satisfying or nourishing. It's not a matter of *if* your body will break down from junk food; it's more a matter of *when*.

There's also the scientifically proven connection between sugar (and all processed carbs that turn to sugar) and diabetes.

Diabetes

Another factor to consider when consuming sugar or processed carbs is the body's insulin response. Sugar doesn't cause diabetes by itself, but consuming lots of added sugar and processed carbohydrates will pave the way. Too much of anything, including sugar, can pack on pounds, for one thing. Heavy bodies have a harder time using and staying sensitive to insulin, the hormone that controls blood sugar. When your body resists insulin, your blood sugar levels and risk of diabetes go sky high.

When we eat or drink sugar, our body releases insulin to help balance our blood sugar. When we overconsume sugar, the pancreas (organ that produces insulin) has two responses:

1. Gets tired and begins to wear out (nontechnical terms) or becomes insulin resistant. This is also known as prediabetes. At this point, the damaging effects of diabetes can usually be reversed with proper nutrition! If an individual does not significantly reduce his or her sugar and processed carb intake (or foods that turn into sugar), diabetes is almost unavoidable.

2. When the pancreas is worn out, then comes type 2 diabetes, or insulin dependency. Paying for and becoming dependent on medication for the rest of your life is expensive and cumbersome and avoidable.

Type 1 diabetes is different. Type 1 diabetes occurs when the body does not produce insulin and is usually diagnosed in children. According to the American Diabetes Association, only 5 percent of all diabetes cases are from type 1; the remaining 95 percent of people with diabetes have type 2.

Our bodies were designed for balanced nutrition. Long-term abuse of any substance will have a negative effect on our bodies. Processed sugar, the sparkling white poison, is one of the worst food substances to abuse.

The Hormone Rollercoaster . . . Leads to Diabetes

As previously stated, too much sugar and too many processed carbohydrates cause a roller coaster of insulin and glucagon (two hormones that regulate our appetite and weight). The first image below demonstrates what happens when we consume too much added sugar or processed carbs in one sitting. Our blood sugar spikes and crashes, unable to stay in the balance zone. The second image reflects a slower rise and fall of the blood sugar, one that keeps the body in balance.

Unhealthy Blood Sugar Pattern

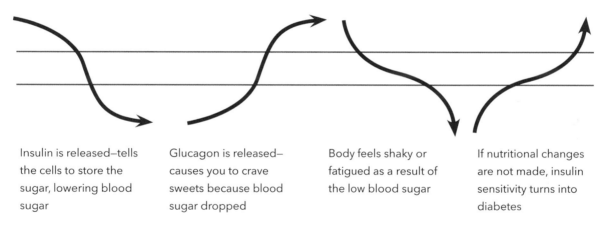

Insulin is released—tells the cells to store the sugar, lowering blood sugar

Glucagon is released—causes you to crave sweets because blood sugar dropped

Body feels shaky or fatigued as a result of the low blood sugar

If nutritional changes are not made, insulin sensitivity turns into diabetes

Healthy Blood Sugar Pattern

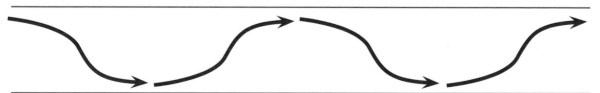

Eating is as much an art as it is a science. To stay within your healthy blood sugar balance, listen to how your body feels after you eat. Are you hungry within one hour of eating? Are you shaky if you wait too long? Are you tired in the midafternoon? Unsatisfied? You will be satisfied and energized by staying within a healthy blood sugar range. Eating whole foods, healthy fats, and proteins at regular intervals are must-haves for feeling great and maintaining a healthy weight.

Effect of Sugar and Processed Food on Children

Whether or not you have children, you will likely interact with a child at some point. Do not think you are giving them a reward by constantly feeding them snacks and candy with added sugar. You are "spoiling" them—but not in the way you may be intending. Instead, offer your time and attention as a gift—this is what children treasure more than anything. Reserve treats for special occasions like birthdays and graduations. Be known as the grandparent who takes the kids to the park, or the aunt who colors, or the in-law who takes them camping or fishing. Create memories with kids, not sugar addictions.

Children are also negatively affected when consuming sugar and processed foods. Like adults, when children consume sugar, their blood sugar rises and their little bodies produce insulin, which drives the blood sugar down too fast, causing:

- Obesity
- Brain fog
- Irritability and tantrums
- Hunger headaches
- Sugar cravings
- Sleep disturbances

Say *No Thank You* to Added Sugar and Processed Foods

My children behave better when we say *no thank you* to added sugar, artificial sugar, and processed carbs. Instead, we enjoy natural desserts like our favorite fruits, chemical-free ice cream and dark chocolate, and homemade treats sweetened with coconut, real cocoa, honey, and maple syrup. Saying a firm no to children when it comes to added sugar can be challenging at first (as adults, we know this struggle, right?), but *no* is the right word to say. Also, try phrases like:

- I'm going to slice up some fresh strawberries for you instead.
- What's your favorite fruit? I'll pick that up the next time I'm at the store.
- How about a square of dark chocolate instead? (And then be sure to put the rest away.)

Avoiding added sugar is especially important for children (and adults) with ADHD and autism. Because sugar affects our brains, the negative side effects are magnified for children with brain disorders.

The more sugar we eat, the more we crave. This cycle is true for children as well. Developing good habits with our families is challenging when everyone else gives in to the no-rules-apply attitude toward sugar. I challenge you to take the path less traveled and watch the benefits unfold. Like anything worthwhile, better health takes time and discipline. Practicing better choices will help keep brain health on the top of your priority list.

Summing up this monumental discovery, less added sugar equals less disease.

Do not be tricked into thinking you can swap sugar with artificial sweeteners to avoid consequences.

Artificial Sweeteners

Artificial sweeteners like sucralose, aspartame (NutraSweet), and Splenda cause real damage to your metabolism and your brain! Studies have shown that people who drink diet soda on a regular basis consume more calories in a day than those who drink regular soda or none at all.

Additionally, the artificial sweetener aspartame (NutraSweet) is an excitotoxin, a chemical suggested to cause permanent damage to your brain's appetite control center.

How Much Sugar Do You *Need*?

Would you be surprised to learn that not one single function in the entire body depends on refined sugar or processed carbohydrates? In fact, you can train your taste buds to enjoy things that aren't as sweet. Try cutting out one sweet food from your diet each day. For example, pass on dessert after dinner. Slowly reduce the sugar in your coffee or change your breakfast. Over time, your physical craving will lessen for that sugar taste.

John 10:10 states: "The thief comes only to steal and kill and destroy; I have come that they may have life, and have it to the full." All the listed consequences of addiction lead to death, not life. Are you willing to continue your negative habits just because everyone else does? Because they are socially acceptable? Because you haven't been diagnosed with a life-threatening disease yet?

Friends, it's time to make some changes in our nutrition habits and be responsible, disciplined stewards of everything we put in our bodies. Change is not as daunting as you think. Start small.

Is your weight something you have battled with for a long time? Maybe even your whole life? If so, use this space to write a prayer to God, giving him your struggles. Listen for and trust the guidance of the Holy Spirit in this area of your life.

_____

_____

_____

_____

_____

_____

_____

_____

_____

_____

_____

_____

_____

_____

_____

_____

Practice

Read labels this week. Count how many grams of sugar are in each food and beverage you consume. Keep track for three days and record it in the reflection section in day 7.

Week 3, Day 5: There Is Hope!

Today, Dawn desires to share more of her personal journey to encourage you in your pursuit of abundant life. In the story below, she unfolds a tangled web of family struggle, sugar addiction, and finding hope.

> Growing up in an abusive family was traumatizing. I never felt safe. I had a pit of loneliness deep down in my stomach. I was only six years old when I first remember my dad beating my mom in the closet. I would hide under my bed and eat frosting right out of the can.
>
> As I got older, I used to gulp down a Diet Coke every morning to try to fill the hole in my stomach. It never worked—the caffeine gave me brief bouts of energy, but in return, the soda messed up my adrenal glands, stress hormones, and sleep cycles. I would also gulp down bagels and Subway sandwiches, thinking I was eating healthily.
>
> As I grew into my midtwenties and thirties, I had three things I ran to before God, also known as idols: sugar, Diet Coke, and excessive work. As I got older, it was easier for me to be a good student, go to college, and work obsessively instead of being present with my immediate family. None of my family members or brothers and sisters truly loved me; I was only used as a pawn in my father's manipulative games to control people with money.
>
> I used idols instead of turning to God. It's not that I didn't grow up with faith in my life—I attended confirmation with my friends the Schweigerts, and my grandma Lynette sang "This Little Light of Mine" to me as a child.
>
> In 2009, I truly found God's love through Westbridge Church, and my entire life has been transformed. The transformation started by simply learning about God and his love, praying nightly, and having the courage to make changes in my life.
>
> I have since made many changes in my spiritual, emotional, and physical health. I am delighted to say that I'm *no longer addicted to sugar*. I know what to eat now to *nourish* my body instead of just fuel it. I gave up Diet Coke in 2015 and acquired a new fondness for hot tea and water. Over the last several years, I have no longer worked excessively. I left my stressful job, spent balanced time with my three beautiful kids, and took health and wellness classes, and now I enjoy spending daily time with many new friends and God.
>
> God gave me a new life, one filled with abundance. There is hope for you too, friend.

There is always hope. Jesus is our hope and our strength. There is hope for you, and there is hope for me. God can and will break us free from our struggles and addictions. We need to be willing to roll our sleeves up and do some work, creating systems and boundaries to keep our intentions successful.

To tackle food addictions, let's look first in the pantry.

Remember the FOSS chart? It may be time for an extreme pantry makeover!

1. Get rid of all table sugar (white granulated stuff)
2. Get rid of processed, enriched, or all-purpose flour
3. Get rid of all packaged food with sugar and/or flour ingredients found in the "processed" column of the FOSS chart.

What should fill your pantry and fridge?

1. Organic cane sugar, unrefined sugar, real maple syrup, and honey
2. Organic wheat flour; gluten-free flours, such as almond and coconut flour
3. Find packaged foods with natural and unprocessed sugar and 100 percent whole-grain or gluten-free flour

The reason I'm not recommending specific brands is because sometimes the company gets purchased by another, larger company. To save costs, the larger company may use cheaper ingredients. Sadly, I have seen this happen to a few of my favorite brands. Read labels.

What Else Can Replace Sugar and Processed Carbs?

Complex Carbs

Carbohydrates come in two main sources—simple and complex—and there are healthy foods in both categories. Complex carbohydrates are more nourishing options than simple carbs with the exception of fruit and raw dairy. Simple carbohydrates are generally responsible for spiking the blood sugar; your body releases insulin as a response when you consume foods that are high in sugar and low or void of natural nutrients and fiber. On the other hand, complex carbohydrates are balanced, nutritious sources that help to regulate our blood sugar and load us up with vital nutrients. Some examples of complex carbohydrates include:

- Vegetables
- Nuts and seeds
- Legumes
- Potatoes
- Black beans
- Quinoa

- Sweet potatoes
- Acorn squash
- Barley
- Green peas
- Oatmeal
- 100 percent whole grains (if it doesn't say 100 percent on the label, it only needs to contain 51 percent whole grains to get the "whole grain" classification)

When it comes to choosing carbohydrates, vegetables should be your first choice!

Gluten-Free Grains?

Do you need to go gluten-free? How do you know? What is gluten?

Gluten is a protein found in the grains of wheat, barley, and rye. Think of gluten as the glue that holds grains together and gives them a nice texture and smooth flavor. There is nothing inherently harmful with gluten. However, some people become sensitive to gluten as a result of:

- Overeating gluten
- Eating grains that are genetically modified
- Intestinal tract issues

The two types of people who should not eat gluten include:

1. Individuals who have a sensitivity to and become ill after eating gluten (e.g., after eating grains, there is an onset of an upset stomach, gas, and bloating). Some experience a flare-up in skin conditions like rosacea and dermatitis. Fortunately, these annoying side effects of eating grains do not usually cause permanent damage, and they go away once you stop eating gluten.

2. Individuals who have a severe condition called celiac disease or many other autoimmune disorders such as Hashimoto's thyroiditis or lupus. Celiac disease results in damage to the intestines, gastrointestinal distress, and nutritional deficiencies. If left untreated, these reactions can lead to intestinal cancers, osteoporosis, and infertility. An *Archives of Internal Medicine* study in 2003 suggests that celiac disease is far more prevalent than anyone has suspected, affecting 1 in 133 Americans.

If you get ill after eating gluten or other grains—or you suspect you may have celiac disease or another autoimmune disease, stop eating grains and consult with your physician.

Some people still get an upset stomach after eating grains even if they are not gluten intolerant or suffering from celiac disease. This uncomfortable condition could be due to your body not breaking down the grain or absorbing all the nutrients properly. If I am describing you, try eating sprouted or fermented grains (we'll look at fermented grains in week 6).

Why Should Grains and Legumes Be Soaked or Sprouted?

Think of grains like chicken eggs. There is a hard shell on the outside to protect the goodness on the inside. The shell is an obvious barrier to the nutrients inside. Most of our grains have a similar shell that contains an antinutrient called phytic acid. Phytic acid acts as a barrier to protect the natural goodness inside the grain.

Think of the elements in nature that the grain or seed must go through to be scattered onto the ground, dug down into the earth, and then sprout before it becomes a strong plant or vegetable. This barrier on the grain is natural protection. While this is good for the grains,

MINDFULNESS

MINDFULNESS

preservation of the shell barrier is not so useful for our bodies—so we should soak the seeds, grains, and legumes before they are cooked or baked and eaten.

When grains and seeds are soaked or sprouted, the natural shells breaks down, and the phytic acid levels are lowered, allowing your body to absorb more of the nutrients available in the grain. If you have never tried sprouted or soaked seeds, grains, or legumes, I strongly encourage you to taste them! Companies who manufacture sprouted or soaked grains are proud to display this healthy method which they do to ensure you receive the most nutrients possible. Sprouting and soaking takes time, but the benefits far outweigh the time it takes to produce essential nutrients.

Soaked Grains, Seeds, and Legumes

Our ancestors have been soaking and sprouting foods for thousands of years, and the evidence coming out is increasingly in favor of sprouting. Sprouting grains increases the absorption of many of the essential nutrients, including B vitamins, vitamin C, folate, fiber, and essential amino acids, such as lysine, which is often lacking in processed grains. Many individuals who are not gluten intolerant but still get ill after eating grains switch to sprouted or soaked grains and are pleasantly surprised to feel great, stay satisfied longer, and have better digestion! Recent demand for convenience foods, however, has caused companies to neglect this ancient tradition. Soaking phytate-rich foods is not a quick process, but once you get into a routine, soaking brown rice, almonds, beans, and other foods becomes habit. The health benefits are worth the effort.

I recommend replacing your white flour and whole grains with sprouted grain products whenever possible. Food for Life and TruRoots are among a few brands that offer a wonderful variety of sprouted products. But remember, read labels. Brands may change ingredients.

Here are just a few more proven reasons to switch to soaked or sprouted grains today:

According to the Westin A. Price Foundation, "Studies on phytic acid reveal that for some people, the phytic acid in whole grains blocks calcium, zinc, magnesium, iron and copper; others seem immune to these adverse consequences, probably because of favorable gut flora, which in some cases can break down phytic acid. In addition, when animal fats providing vitamins A and D accompany dietary whole grains, the effects of phytic acid are mitigated."

The foundation goes on to recommend no more than two to three servings per day of phytate-rich foods. "Daily consumption of one or two slices of genuine sourdough bread, a handful of nuts, and one serving of properly prepared oatmeal, pancakes, brown rice or beans should not pose any problems in the

Rather than allowing yourself to fall into the mind-set of, "Is this food good or bad?" make your choices based on, "What is my best option in the given situation?"

context of a nutrient-dense diet. Problems arise when whole grains and beans become the major dietary sources of calories—when every meal contains more than one whole grain product or when over-reliance is placed on nuts or legumes." Remember, our health choices fall on a continuum. Rather than allowing yourself to fall into the mind-set of, *"Is this food good or bad?"* make your choices based on, *"What is my best option in the given situation?"* When in doubt, reference the FOSS Chart and make your best choice.

Full disclosure: I purchase products that use sprouted grains, but I do not *sprout* my own grains, yet. However, I *do* take the time to *soak* most seeds, beans, grains, and legumes. I started with organic brown rice, which was the easiest for me to soak overnight in salt water and then cook the next day. Once I was comfortable with brown rice, I started soaking almonds overnight in salt water. Then came oats (my son *loves* the taste of soaked and cooked oats), beans, and seeds. I had to throw out a few batches due to forgetting about the jar . . . but overall, I am pleased with the result of taste, texture, and better absorption due to soaking phytate-rich foods.

Seeds Are for More Than Just the Birds

Seeds like quinoa and chia are high in fiber, antioxidants, and protein. Chia is also high in omega-3s.

Some additional seeds that I keep on hand are pumpkin and sunflower seeds, and buckwheat. Soaked and dehydrated seeds are best. Seeds can be eaten plain or used in:

- Yogurt
- Cereal
- Smoothies
- Salads
- Baked goods

The recommended serving size for most seeds is two tablespoons.

In Summary, Select Unprocessed Grains

The challenge of selecting carbs is eating against the grain (choosing whole, sprouted grains over processed, refined grains). And the enjoyable part of my job is watching the transformation of those individuals who reduce their processed and enriched grain and sugar intake. Check out the FOSS chart to make your best choice when selecting flour and grains.

FOSS	Processed Food (Toxic)—Avoid	Less Processed (Some Health Benefits)	Unprocessed (Nourishing)— Enjoy in Moderation	Enjoy with Reckless Abandon
Flour & Grains	Enriched flour Bleached flour Bulgur White flour products Puffed grain products, such as rice cakes Factory-made modern soy foods Soybeans, unless used for making fermented foods like natto Soybean sprouting seeds and sprouts Alfalfa seeds and sprouts	100 percent whole grains Unsoaked granola Dried beans and lentils Unsoaked whole-grain rice Canned beans Buckwheat, corn, and brown rice pasta Organic white rice	Soaked and/or sprouted grains; fermented grains, such as sourdough Organic dried beans and lentils Soaked and/or sprouted 100 percent whole grains and whole-grain break-fast cereals that must be cooked Wild rice Organic popcorn (to pop at home) Organic sprouting seeds except alfalfa and soybean	Nothing except the love of Jesus!

Consuming unprocessed foods has a number of sweet benefits:

- Less inflammation in the body—Less pain in the muscles, joints, and bones (think about arthritis—which is inflammation in the joints). Imagine waking up in the morning with less pain.

- Weight loss—This one may seem obvious, but we often don't realize how much easier it is to lose weight when we aren't battling our own hormones. I do not know how else to convince you but to beg you to reduce your consumption of added sugar and processed carbs and see the benefits for yourself. If you try nothing else with carbohydrate adjustments, try avoiding treats for a week and make informed choices with processed carbohydrates based on how you feel after that week.

- Reduced craving for sugar—Over time (usually around two weeks), our bodies stop craving added sugar and start craving and having more enjoyment of natural sugars in fruits and vegetables.

- Healthy insulin response—Your organs will be able to respond to the healthy sugars in fruits, vegetables, and dairy without getting stressed.

Week 3, Day 6: The Sugar-Free Challenge

Now that you've learned about sugar and processed carbs, start thinking about taking a break (fast) from them! Next week, we're going to implement the sugar-free challenge with a partner. But if you start thinking about the challenge now and prepping your pantry, you'll set yourself up for success!

Below are a few examples of how you could swap out your high-sugar meals and snacks with some low- to no-sugar options.

The sugar count in the charts below excludes naturally occurring sugar found in fruits, vegetables, and dairy.

You Have Options

Breakfast

Avoid	Try Instead
Cereal and milk and lite mocha from coffee shop	1 hard-boiled egg, half of an orange, and green tea from coffee shop
Added sugar: *approximately 51 grams*	**Added sugar:** *0 grams*

Lunch

Avoid	Try Instead
White bread sandwich with deli meat, mayo, and 12-ounce soda	Salad with grilled chicken, extra-virgin olive oil, avocado, cheese, nuts, and 20 ounces sparkling water
Added sugar: *approximately 56 grams*	**Added sugar:** *0 grams*

Snack

Avoid	Try Instead
Protein bar and chocolate milk	Gas station apple and cheese stick
Added sugar: *approximately 67 grams*	**Added sugar:** *0 grams*

Dinner

Avoid	Try Instead
Restaurant burger, fries, and small milkshake	Restaurant veggie stir-fry with lean beef or chicken and fresh fruit and cheese for dessert
Added sugar: *approximately 164 grams*	**Added sugar:** *0 grams*

Dessert

Avoid	Try Instead
Big bowl of ice cream	Single serving of frozen banana "ice cream"* (See page 134 for recipe.)
Added sugar: *approximately 54 grams*	**Added sugar:** *0 grams*

Avoid this total: 392 grams (1,568 calories in sugar)
Try this instead: 0 grams

The "avoid this" columns contain more than ten times the recommended daily total for added sugar.

Go take thirty-one tablespoons of sugar, put it in a glass or bowl, and think about eating it (but do not eat it!). Do this exercise with children if you have them in the house.

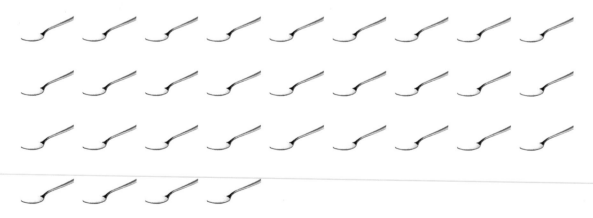

Do you know how much exercise is needed to burn all that sugar *from just one day*?

15.68 hours of walking

5.22 hours of strength training

3.14 hours of running

The above sugar-filled day is a realistic tragedy for many Americans. "Avoid this" is what my day could have looked like before I realized God actually cared about my physical health and well-being. I was tired, my allergies were terrible, I had adult acne, and I got stomachaches often. There should be no wonder why Americans suffer from so much chronic pain, obesity, and disease.

We must recognize the seriousness of our excessive sugar and processed carb intake. The mind-set of "I have a sweet tooth and there is nothing I can do about my cravings" is not a harmless excuse. Sugar and processed foods are killing us, and addictions are getting worse with more and more convenience foods added to the market. Now is the time to make changes in our thinking and in our actions. Now is the time to be sick and tired of being sick and tired! Let's say NO MORE to chronic pain, depression, anxiety, bottomless cravings, roller-coastering weight, daily fatigue, and disease.

> *You are the only one who can make the decision to become the person you were created to be.*

You can do something about your health! You can take charge of your health. Small changes lead to a lifetime of healthier decisions. *You are the only one who can make the decision to become the person you were created to be.*

What commitment will you make today to replace processed food with real food?

_____

_____

_____

How do you think your health will improve?

_____

_____

_____

You can do it!

Do you know how much added sugar you need per day to be healthy? If you said zero grams, you are correct.

*Banana Ice Cream Recipe, Grams of Added Sugar: ZERO

Ingredients
1 ripe banana

Directions
Peel one banana and cut it up into chunks. Put the chunks into a freezer-safe container and freeze. Take banana chunks out of freezer and let sit out for 10 minutes. Put chunks in a high-powered blender or food processer and blend until smooth. Enjoy!

Feel free to add frozen strawberries, nut butter, pecans, or any healthy flavors to your "ice cream!"

Week 3, Day 7: Recap & Reflect

Should you avoid added sugar and processed carbohydrates? Yes.

When I encourage participants to avoid sugar and processed carbs, the panicked question inevitably arises, "What am I going to eat? What am I going to do without my sugary cereal in the morning, white bread at lunch, or sweet treats during holidays?"

My job becomes fun and challenging at this point. Refer back to weeks 2 and 3; I listed dozens of protein sources, delicious protein-packed recipes, and ninety-eight fruits and vegetables available at most grocery stores! There are so many healthy foods you can eat without consuming excessive added sugar and processed carbohydrates. As you may have discovered, changing your eating habits takes time, and it will certainly be challenging, but trust me when I say change is possible. You can do it! You are worth the challenge. Your palate will change. Eventually (if you are not already there), you will like—and dare I say *crave*?—whole foods over junk food!

- The American Heart Association recommends that men limit added sugar to 36 grams, or 9 teaspoons, per day and that women limit added sugar to 24 grams, or 6 teaspoons, per day. This does not include fruit, vegetable, and dairy sugar, which are balanced with nutrients, fiber, and/or protein. Of all the calories consumed daily, a maximum of 10 percent should come from added sugar, according to the 2015 USDA guidelines. This marks a dramatic reduction from 25 percent since the last USDA recommendation. Remember that despite these guidelines, your body does not require *any* added sugar.

- There are dozens of books on the shelves highlighting the dangerous effects of sugar. Yet the danger of sugar is such an unpopular topic. Is it because we're all addicted? Yes. We must reduce our sugar from processed carbs, packaged foods, and sweets, and increase our servings of vegetables, fruits, fat, and whole grains. Our lives depend on it. The quality of *your* life depends on it.

- The easiest way to reduce your sugar and processed carb cravings is to make small daily efforts to reduce your consumption. Be cautious not to replace sugar with artificial sweeteners. Instead, replace your sugary and processed foods with natural sweeteners such as organic cane sugar, real honey and maple syrup, organic blue agave, liquid stevia, and fruit.

- The majority of your complex carbohydrate consumption should be from vegetables.

How you feel today is the culmination of everything you ate and drank, how much you moved, and how well you slept the past three days.

Practice

Keep track of your sugar grams here:

Day 1 _____ Sugar grams

Day 2 _____ Sugar grams

Day 3 _____ Sugar grams

What surprised you about your sugar consumption?

_____

_____

_____

Did you make any immediate changes as a result of this experiment? Y/N

If yes, what changes did you make?

_____

_____

_____

Have you invited God into your health journey yet? yes/no

_____

_____

If so, write about that experience.

_____

_____

_____

_____

_____

Reflection Notes:

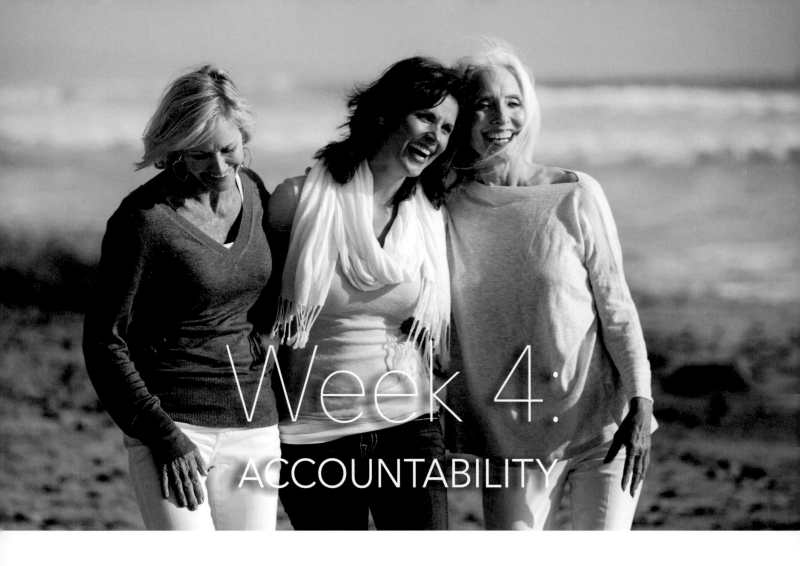

Week 4:
ACCOUNTABILITY

Welcome to week 4!

Moving along with the five keys to success, we will continue thinking about the role of accountability in our long-term success. Are you continuing to touch base with a check-in partner daily? Are you still writing in your journal? Staying accountable to yourself, others, and God makes the journey more enjoyable and successful.

**As iron sharpens iron,
so one person sharpens another.**

- Proverbs 27:17

Week 4 Action Steps

Number one health goal: _____ *Goal Accomplished!* ☐

Accountability

Record your **strength** workouts in the *Living Wellness Journal*;

weekly goal:_____ _____ (number of days) (minutes per day) ☐

  Partner's goal: _____ _____ (number of days) (minutes per day)

Record your **cardio** workouts in the *Living Wellness Journal*;

weekly goal:_____ _____ (number of days) (minutes per day) ☐

  Partner's goal: _____ _____ ☐

What is your **nutrition** goal this week (remember the SMART goals)? Sugar Challenge ☐
☐ ☐ ☐ ☐ ☐ ☐

  Partner's nutrition goal: Sugar Challenge or other: _____

Record your **food/beverage** intake in *Living Wellness Journal* or app ☐

Check in with your partner daily. ☐ ☐ ☐ ☐ ☐ ☐ ☐

Knowledge

Read and fill out all questions in this book prior to the next meeting. ☐

Mindfulness

Read labels to identify trans fats and partially hydrogenated fats in packaged and processed foods and cooking oils. ☐

Inspiration

Ask God to reveal any false truths you may believe about your body image. Then ask for God to reveal his truth to you. ☐

Motivation

Why is it so easy to spend money on our toys, hobbies, children, or pets but not on our own preventative health measures? List one cost-effective investment you will make into your health this week: _____ ☐

Living Wellness Week 4 Exercises

Add these two exercises to your existing strength training routine.

Prone Plank

Begin in tabletop position (hands and knees). You can maintain tabletop posture or make the exercise more difficult by dropping down to your elbows and moving your knees in a position that straightens your back (as shown in Option I). Pull your belly button into your spine and tighten your butt muscles. Avoid an excessive arch in your low back. If this causes any pain in your back or shoulders, stop immediately.

For option II, lift off your knees into a full-body plank.

Breathe while you hold your posture for thirty seconds to one minute. Repeat as time permits.

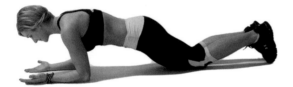

Option I

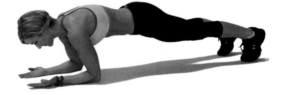

Option II

Stability Ball Hamstring Curls

Lie on your back and place a stability (exercise) ball under your feet and calves. Inhale as you lift your hips off the ground with straight legs. Exhale as you keep your hips off the ground and bend your knees toward your body.

For Option II, lift one leg straight in the air as you bend your knee toward your body.

Perform 16 to 20 reps or 8 to 10 reps each of the single-leg hamstring curls. Repeat as time permits. Do these exercises every other day. Remember to stretch your muscles after your workout.

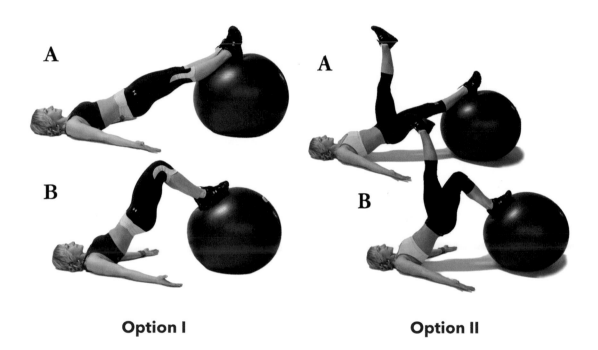

Option I　　　　　　　　　　**Option II**

Sugar Challenge*

1. Select a number of days to take the Sugar Challenge (1-7 days)
   _____

2. Select a target number of grams to stay under for those days (remember, zero grams is an option) _____ sugar grams to stay under

3. Record your sugar grams here:

Day	Goal	Actual
1		
2		
3		
4		
5		
6		
7		

* If you want to take this challenge to the next level, eliminate processed carbs as well!

Looking Ahead

This week, we get to implement the sugar challenge. We'll also learn about dietary fat, one of the most important topics in the whole book.

Week 4, Day 2: Macronutrient – Fat
One of the most important nutrition topics in this book

Because healthy fat consumption is so satisfying, fat is one of my favorite topics in nutrition. It was probably one of my least favorites when I was overweight and unhealthy, but that is in my past, and fat is a vital health topic, so let's examine it together.

Consuming dietary fat does not make you fat. No. Fat does not make you fat, and if you argue with me, you will see I am passionate to share the good news I have discovered: dietary fat is vital to exceptional health.

An excess of dietary fat *can* lead to an increase of body fat (adipose tissue). Guess what? The excess of any calorie, regardless of where it comes from, leads to an increase in body fat. Remember, food is energy. If calories do not get used, they get stored!

Dietary fat plays a vital role in:

- Brain and organ function
- Digestion
- Vitamin and mineral absorption
- Nerve health
- Maintaining a healthy body weight

Look at that list! We need to consume fat to be healthy! "But, Ashley, vital fat does not make me look better in my bathing suit," you might say. Our industrialized diets have caused a dangerous shift toward us becoming a fat-free nation, based on the myth that eating fat makes us fat and increases our cholesterol levels.

Eating fat-free often leads to an increase in sodium, sugar, chemical additives, and/or refined grains in foods to make up for lost flavor and texture. Go back with me to high school biology. Which vitamins are fat-soluble? Right! A, D, E, and K. What does that mean? Fat-soluble means that you need to consume dietary fat for your body to break down and absorb the vitamins. If you are not getting enough healthy dietary fat, you are not absorbing vital nutrients.

Tell me, has there been an equally rising correlation between the deficiency of vitamins A and D as our diets shift toward fat-free? The answer is absolutely yes, and the symptoms are evident.

One of my favorite nutritionists and authors, Jonny Bowden, lists avocados (containing all three healthy sources of fat) as an outstanding choice for healthy fat in his book *The 150 Healthiest Foods on Earth.* Participants ask me if they should skip adding avocados or olive oil to their salads to cut calories. The answer every time is: *No*, do not compromise your health by skipping fats to make a calorie deficit. Instead, avoid refined grains, added sugar, and liquids (other than water) as a means of cutting unnecessary calories. Any extreme shift in nutrition on either side of excess or deficit is dangerous because our bodies were and are still designed for balance. Most fats are healthy in the proper proportions. Some are unhealthy altogether.

Four Types of Fat

Trans Fatty Acids (Trans Fats) ***Run for your life from this one***

• Partially hydrogenated oils

Saturated Fatty Acids (Saturated Fats)

• Animal fat: eggs, butter, cheese, milk, lard, and tallow

• Tropical oils: coconut and palm oil

Monounsaturated Fatty Acids (Unsaturated Fats)

• Olive oil, nuts, high-oleic safflower oil, sunflower oil, avocados and avocado oil, vegetable oil (not recommended), and canola oil (not recommended)

Polyunsaturated Fatty Acids (Unsaturated Fats)

• Omega-3s: fish oil, walnuts, flaxseed, soybean oil (not recommended), and canola oil (not recommended)

• Omega-6s: vegetable oils like safflower, corn oil (not recommended), and soybean oil (not recommended)

We will dive deep into each type of fat this week. Take a look in your pantry and see what kind of fats and oils you have. Start becoming emotionally detached from your unhealthy oils so that when I ask you to throw them away and replace them with nourishing oils, you will be ready.

For today, spend some time thinking about your past and current relationship with dietary fat.

What do you believe to be true about consuming dietary fat?

WEEK 4

144 LIVING WELLNESS FOR GROWTH GROUPS

How would changing your thoughts about fat lead to a healthier lifestyle?

_____

_____

_____

_____

What kinds of oils and fats are in your pantry?

_____

_____

_____

_____

Week 4, Day 3: Not All Fats Are Created Equal

Oils and fats are big business. The chemistry and processing of oils are complicated, but there are a few key factors to keep in mind when selecting oils and fats. Let's take a look at part of the FOSS chart highlighting oils and fats before we dive into the details.

FOSS	Processed Food (Toxic)–Avoid	Less Processed (Some Health Benefits)	Unprocessed (Nourishing)– Enjoy in Moderation	Enjoy with Reckless Abandon
Oils & Fats	Partially hydrogenated oils Most commercial vegetable oils, including cottonseed, soy, corn, canola, rice bran, hemp, and grapeseed oils All margarines, spreads, and partially hydrogenated vegetable shortenings	Pasteurized grass-fed butter Cold-pressed or expeller-pressed sesame, sunflower, peanut, macadamia, avocado, almond, walnut, pecan, pistachio, hazelnut, pumpkin seed, and high-oleic safflower oils in small amounts Refined palm oil Refined coconut oil Extra-virgin olive oil Cold-pressed flaxseed oil	Raw grass-fed butter, organic cold-pressed flaxseed oil, extra-virgin sesame oil, red palm oil Organic extra-virgin olive oil Organic cold-pressed macadamia, avocado, almond, high-oleic sunflower, and high-oleic safflower oils Organic unrefined virgin coconut oil Unrefined organic palm oil Fat and lard from pigs allowed to graze Tallow and suet from grass-fed cows and sheep Poultry fat from pastured poultry	It's a fallacy that you can eat endless amounts of anything.

Three Main Types of Oil Extraction

Cooking oils come from seeds, nuts, and/or fruit. Imagine the oil in one of your bottles on the shelf. How do you suppose the oil got from the seed, nut, or fruit into the bottle? There are no liquid oil trees that we can stick a tap in to get a substance like maple syrup. The oil must be extracted in order for us to use it for cooking and baking. The extraction process either preserves the goodness and nourishment in the oil or the process damages the oil and makes it toxic and rancid.

1. **Cold-Pressed, Unrefined ~ This is the Good Stuff**

Cold-pressed, unrefined oils are worth their weight in gold. These oils contain a plethora of essential nutrients for our bodies and brains. You'll read more this week about the benefits of healthy dietary fat, but for now, when purchasing most *liquid* oils, look for the words *cold-pressed*, *unrefined*, and *organic*. Your body will thank you!

2. **Expeller-Pressed ~ Some Bad, Some Good**

Many years ago, extraction happened by slow-moving stone expeller presses. The process was time consuming, but it protected the integrity of the oil by keeping the temperature low and the light exposure minimal. Like most of the food industry, small processing factories were bought up by huge factories looking for ways to speed up the extraction process and save money. I don't think big food companies set out to slowly kill us by producing toxic oils, but I think short-term greed gets in the way of looking at long-term health consequences. The problem with crushing seeds, nuts, and fruit in huge machines is that it introduces a tremendous amount of heat. Read the quote below from leading researcher Mary Enig on the effects of high heat processing:

"High-temperature processing causes the weak carbon bonds of unsaturated fatty acids, especially triple unsaturated linolenic acid, to break apart, thereby creating dangerous free radicals. In addition, antioxidants such as fat-soluble vitamin E, which protect the body from the ravages of free radicals, are neutralized or destroyed by high temperatures and pressures. BHT and BHA, both suspected of causing cancer and brain damage, are often added to these oils to replace vitamin E and other natural preservatives destroyed by heat." Previously we looked at ingredients to avoid. BHT and BHA are preservatives that are toxic to the body.

Certain oils below are among the most common negatively affected by modern high-heat processing.

Oils That Should Not Be Consumed as Expeller Pressed:

- Corn
- Soybean
- Cottonseed
- Canola (rapeseed)
- Flax (this oil may be safely consumed as a cold-pressed, organic oil)

These oils become rancid in the extraction process, so oftentimes they are put through another process called "deodorizing" to get rid of the rancid smell and taste! Your oil should not need to be deodorized like a smelly armpit in order to be sold and consumed.

Enig goes on to say that "there is a safe modern technique for extraction that drills into the seeds and extracts the oil and its precious cargo of antioxidants under low temperatures, with minimal exposure to light and oxygen. These expeller-expressed, unrefined oils will remain fresh for a long time if stored in the refrigerator in dark bottles. Extra-virgin olive oil is produced by crushing olives between stone or steel rollers. This process is a gentle one that preserves the integrity of the fatty acids and the numerous natural preservatives in olive oil. If olive oil is packaged in opaque containers, it will retain its freshness and precious store of antioxidants for many years."

Some seeds and fruits are safely expeller pressed without causing any damage to the final product.

Expeller-Pressed Oils That Are Safe to Consume:

- Safflower oil
- Sunflower oil
- Sesame seed oils
- Coconut oil
- Palm oil

3. **Chemically Extracted—Avoid**

After the seed, nut, or fruits have been pressed, the last remaining oil is usually chemically extracted with a solvent such as hexane. Although the solvent is boiled off, "up to 100 parts per million may remain in the oil. Such solvents, themselves toxic, also retain the toxic pesticides adhering to seeds and grains before processing begins," says Enig.

Chemically extracted oils are usually the cheapest ones on the shelf, contain the least amount of nutrients and the most chemicals, and should be avoided at all cost.

Another Way Oils Become Damaged

Extraction is not the only way to ruin oil. Another way is by adding hydrogen to the oil as a preservative. You'll read this on the label as:

Partially hydrogenated oils, also known as trans-fatty acids (trans fats).

Oils can become trans fatty during the process of extraction or preservation, or when turning the liquid oils into a solid. According to Enig, "Altered partially hydrogenated fats made from vegetable oils actually block utilization of essential fatty acids, causing many deleterious effects including":

- Paralysis of the immune system
- Increased blood cholesterol
- Sexual dysfunction

Enig goes on to assert that consumption of hydrogenated fats is associated with:

- Cancer
- Atherosclerosis
- Diabetes
- Obesity
- Immune system dysfunction

- Low-birth-weight babies
- Birth defects
- Decreased visual acuity
- Sterility
- Difficulty in lactation
- Problems with bones and tendons

This is a long list of horrible side effects from trans fats and partially hydrogenated oils! We can avoid these health risks, diseases, and side effects simply by *not eating* highly processed fats and oils. Avoid fried, packaged, processed food, and margarine. Yes, especially margarine.

The Nurses' Health Study found that women who ate one and one-third tablespoons of margarine a day had a 50 percent greater risk of heart disease than women who ate margarine only rarely! If you were eating it before, you probably thought margarine was a healthy alternative to butter. Better alternatives to margarine include butter from organic, grass-fed cows; coconut oil; or extra-virgin olive oil.

Read Labels

How do you know if your favorite baked good contains trans fats? Read the label. If the ingredient list shows partially hydrogenated oils or any of the oils listed in the processed column of the FOSS chart, put down the package and find a better alternative. I label most food ingredients as "better or worse," but when it comes to trans fats and processed oils, they are just *bad*.

Here are some places that partially hydrogenated processed oils like to hide:

- Kids' breakfast cereals
- Fried food
- Snack crackers
- Packaged desserts
- Chips
- Frosting
- Frozen pizzas
- Biscuits

Read the label on your prepacked brownie or pancake mix. Vegetable oils and/or partially hydrogenated oils are sure to be on the list!

Make a point to stop eating trans fats and processed oils and watch your health flourish. We do not need to be scared of dietary fat. We need to be educated so we can make informed decisions. Udo Erasmus, PhD in nutrition, states the matter simply: "Trans fats bring twice as many food additives into our diet as all other food additives from all food sources combined."

Please be aware that packaged and processed foods are *big* business. Manufacturers do not need to admit to adding trans fats to food if it is under 0.5 grams. Does this make you feel safe? It makes me angry. How can we avoid the poison if it's not even on the label? The American Heart Association states that "in November 2013, the United States Food and Drug Administration (FDA) made a preliminary determination that partially hydrogenated oils are no longer Generally Recognized as Safe (GRAS) in human food." The goal is to avoid the danger altogether. When possible, steer clear of packaged, processed, and deep-fried foods.

I can't stress enough how much I have seen participants' health improve when they finally accept the fact that processed foods bring disease and early death and whole foods bring life. What an important lesson we can learn from the health journey of others.

Before we go any further, go to your pantry and assess your fat and oil inventory. Which toxic fats and oils will you throw away and which healthy ones will you keep?

_____

_____

_____

Which fats and oils will you purchase to replace the ones you threw away?

_____

_____

_____

Week 4, Day 4: The Fats Your Body *Needs*

Saturated Fat

Saturated fats get mixed reviews because so many people fear their alleged link to high cholesterol. As with dietary fat, we don't need to fear cholesterol; the truth is that 99 percent of people can safely and effectively control their cholesterol with proper nutrition and exercise. Cholesterol is so important that your body makes around 300 milligrams per day! Because of the needs of *every organ in your body*, 300 milligrams is not enough; you need to consume cholesterol from outside sources to obtain adequate amounts. Animal fats and saturated fats in tropical oils (in measured portions) offer wonderful health benefits and nutrients for your cells. Saturated fats also absorb essential vitamins.

Sources of healthy saturated fats to consume in moderation include eggs, raw milk, hard cheese, grass-fed butter, lard, and unrefined tropical oils like coconut and palm oil. Cooking with and eating small amounts of tropical oils and animal fats has wonderful health properties, flavor, and satiating benefits.

Mono- and Polyunsaturated Fats (Unsaturated Fats)

Mono- and polyunsaturated fats play a vital role in maintaining optimal health as well. Unsaturated fats reduce inflammation, balance cholesterol levels, lower blood pressure, stabilize heart rhythms, and help stabilize blood sugar, which keeps your body feeling full and satisfied after a meal or snack. Approximately 30–45 percent (some researchers even suggest up to 50 percent) of your daily calories should come from fat.

When talking about polyunsaturated fat, we need to pause on omega-3 and -6 fatty acids. Because the majority of Americans don't eat a fish-and-vegetable meal profile, most of us are severely lacking in omega-3s. The consequences are evident. Unlike other nutrients, *our bodies do not produce omega fatty acids*. Therefore, we need to obtain omegas through food and supplementation. Omegas are vital for every function in your body. People who are active need even more omegas to help rebuild and repair cells that have been damaged during exercise. The key to unlocking benefits of omegas is not just how much you consume; the key is in the balance of omega-3s to omega-6s (between 1:1 and 1:4 servings, respectively). Practically, this could look like one serving of fish or walnuts and one serving each of avocado and sunflower seeds in a day.

Omega-3 Fatty Acids (Omega-3s)—These Are Essential

According to the Harvard School of Public Health, "Omega-3 fats have been shown to help prevent heart disease and stroke; may help control lupus, eczema, and rheumatoid arthritis; and may play protective roles in cancer and other conditions."

On its website, the Mayo Clinic has a long list of disease preventions and treatments using omega-3s for the following:

- Coronary heart disease
- High blood pressure
- Hyperlipidemia (triglyceride lowering)
- Rheumatoid arthritis
- Secondary cardiovascular disease prevention
- Abnormal heart rhythms

Another list from the Mayo Clinic shows diseases that may benefit from omega-3 supplementation "but needs more research to confirm the findings":

- Aggression
- Allergies
- Anxiety
- Stiff arteries
- Asthma
- Improved athletic performance
- Bipolar disorder
- Weight loss
- Cancer
- Abnormal heart rhythms
- Heart disease
- Chronic obstructive pulmonary disease (COPD)
- Brain function
- Crohn's disease
- Toxicity
- Dementia
- Depression
- Diabetes
- Menstrual cramps
- Eczema

And the list goes on.

The greatest benefit of consuming omega-3s shows itself in our heart health. The Harvard School of Public Health states "omega-3 fats lower blood pressure and heart rate, improve blood vessel function, and, at higher doses, lower triglycerides and may ease inflammation, which plays a role in the development of atherosclerosis." Most notably, the Harvard School of Public Health cites a large study, known as the GISSI Prevention Trial, that shows that "heart attack survivors who took a 1-gram capsule of omega-3 fats every day for three years were less likely to have a repeat heart attack, stroke, or die of sudden death than those who took a placebo. Notably, the risk of sudden cardiac death was reduced by about *50 percent!* [emphasis mine]."

The federal government's dietary guidelines, released in 2011, suggest daily consumption of both DHA and EPA, two main types of omega-3s.

To get a *minimum* weekly intake of 1,750 milligrams of eicosapentaenoic acid (EPA) and docosahexaenoic acid (DHA), consume two four-ounce portions **per week** of any of the following popular seafood and shellfish (listed below with their approximate total content of EPA and DHA per four-ounce portion):

- Salmon (Atlantic, Chinook, Coho): 1,200–2,400 milligrams

- Anchovies: 2,300–2,400 milligrams

- Bluefin tuna: 1,700 milligrams; yellowfin tuna: 150–350 milligrams; canned: 150–300 milligrams

- Sardines: 1,100–1,600 milligrams

- Trout: 1,000–1,100 milligrams

- Crab: 200–550 milligrams

- Cod: 200 milligrams

- Scallops: 200 milligrams

- Lobsters: 200 milligrams

- Tilapia: 150 milligrams

- Shrimp: 100 milligrams

As usual, variety is key!

How Much Dietary Fat Do You Need?

Approximately 30–50 percent of your daily calories should come from fats. This means that for a 1,200-calorie plan, you should consume about 40–67 grams of healthy fat per day.

For a 1,600-calorie plan, you should consume about 53–89 grams per day. And for a 2,000-calorie plan, you should consume about 66–111 grams of fat per day. If you did not calculate your approximate daily caloric intake, refer back to week 1 for that estimate.

Do You Need an Omega-3 Supplement?

If you do not eat fish at least one to two times per week, you may need an omega-3 supplement; if so, look for one with:

- At least 300 milligrams of DHA
- Vitamin E or other natural preservatives such as rosemary extract
- A source from small, oily fish like anchovy, sardines, or menhaden

You can also get omega-3s from non-fish sources, including flaxseed oil, beans, walnuts, and seeds, and such vegetables as winter squash, broccoli, spinach, and cauliflower.

Fish is the highest source of omega-3s, but the danger of consuming too much (more than one to two servings per week from polluted waters) is toxic heavy metals like mercury and lead in your body. Vegetables, flaxseeds, and walnuts are a great way to supplement your omega-3s if you are not consuming at least two servings of fish per week.

Practice

How many servings of omega-3s did you consume in the last week (e.g., fish, flaxseeds, or walnuts)?

_____ servings of omega-3s

Week 4, Day 5: Omega-6 Fatty Acids (Omega-6s)

Omega-6s should be consumed in *limited* quantities.

Omega-6s are more common in our diets than omega-3s. Some studies suggest we consume more than twenty times the omega-6s than we need! Check the ingredients list of your favorite snack foods and you will likely find soybean oil and corn oil, the two most common sources of omega-6s.

We do need omega-6s for our health; the proper amount helps reduce arthritis, allergies, ADHD, and even diabetes. But the problem is most of us get way more omega-6s than we need due to the heavy influence of soy and corn in our diets. By not getting enough omega-3s and consuming too many omega-6s, our body chemistry revolts (metabolic breakdown).

An excessive amount of omega-6s decreases your immune function, increases heart disease, increases symptoms of arthritis, and promotes unhealthy cell growth (leading to or exacerbating cancers). Are you starting to get the picture?

Remember, the proper ratio for omega-3s to omega-6s is between 1:1 and 1:4, respectively.

We need more omega-3s and fewer omega-6s in our diets. We will accomplish this as we clean up and kick out the majority of packaged and fried foods in our pantries.

Eating a balance of omega-3s and omega-6s boosts your body's ability to fight off the common cold, complex diseases, and keeps lipids (fats) in check in your bloodstream. Consuming a proper balance also leads to a reduction of inflammation in your body.

Inflammation is the number-one source of physical pain in your body and a breeding ground for disease. The balance of omega-3s and omega-6s is especially important if you work out on a regular basis. Imagine pumping thick (full of fat) blood through a weak heart, clogged arteries, and swollen muscles; it looks (sounds?) like an aneurysm. Consuming the right amount of omega-3s and omega-6s (and practicing regular exercise) will keep your body pumping unclogged blood through a strong heart and healthy arteries and veins.

Practice

How many total grams of fat are you consuming per day? Track for one day and record it here:

Dietary Fat _____ grams

Week 4, Day 6: Baking and Cooking with Fats and Oils

Use the guide below when cooking, baking, or frying your foods.

Low heat: Seed oils like flaxseed get damaged and carcinogenic when introduced to high heat. A carcinogenic oil does damage to every cell in the body, increasing aging and the risk of cancer. Instead, steam your veggies with water and drizzle the organic cold-pressed flaxseed oil on top before serving to preserve all the nutrients.

Medium heat: Cooking or baking with butter, tropical oils, and extra-virgin olive oil are good options when using medium heat (e.g., pan frying an egg, baking, or cooking 100 percent whole-grains, or sprouted pasta).

High heat: For high-heat baking, grilling, or frying foods, use saturated fats, such as unrefined coconut, palm oils, lard, or tallow (e.g., frying chicken or steak in lard preserves the nutrients and gives the food a light, delicious flavor without the harmful effects of damaged oil).

Learning and practicing how to use healthy fats to prepare and cook your foods not only removes a significant amount of carcinogens from your diet but also offers rewarding benefits that will affect your health right now in tangible ways (less pain in your joints from inflammation, for instance).

Fat-Friendly Day—Example Ideas

Breakfast:

- Organic raw whole milk or unsweetened coconut milk in your coffee or tea, 1 gram of fat
- ½ tablespoon organic butter on sprouted wheat or sourdough bread, 6 grams of fat
- One pan-fried egg (in butter) with Swiss cheese, 12.5 grams of fat
- 1 orange, 0 grams of fat

Midmorning Snack:

- Homemade fruit smoothie with one serving of coconut milk and/or plain yogurt, 6 grams of fat

Lunch:

- Salad with organic dressing (avoid trans fats) or extra-virgin oil/balsamic vinegar and seasoning, 14 grams of fat

- 1/2 of a small avocado, 10 grams of fat
- 1 serving of protein—chicken, fish, or beans (on the side or on your salad), 4 grams of fat

Midday Snack:

- Organic red pepper slices with guacamole or hummus (read labels to avoid processed oils on the ingredient label), 4 grams of fat
- One glass of kombucha, 0 grams of fat

Dinner:

- Grilled or baked burgers, fish, or steak, 24 grams of fat. (Grilling is controversial because of the possible carcinogenic response from charring your meat. Don't overcook your meat when you grill. Use marinades with spices such as basil, marjoram, mint, oregano, rosemary, sage, and thyme, which are all powerful antioxidants that may combat damage from carcinogens. Avoid marinades that contain added sugar.)
- Variety of steamed and pickled vegetables drizzled with extra-virgin olive oil, 14 grams of fat

Dessert:

- A glass of unsweetened coconut or almond milk and one square of organic dark chocolate, 1 gram of fat

Seasoning Blend Idea (homemade—use within three days):

- Oregano, dill, basil, fresh lemon zest, unsweetened coconut flakes, Celtic sea salt, and pepper. Mix together and sprinkle on veggies, salad, or pasta. 0 grams of fat

Total Fat: 96.5 grams—This is a satisfying and healthy day!

What groceries will you get to increase your healthy fat intake? (i.e. avocados, eggs, grass-fed butter, full-fat yogurt)

Week 4, Day 7: Recap & Reflect

Medical doctors, to whom we have entrusted our health because we have not yet learned to care for it ourselves, studied disease rather than health in medical school. Their curriculum included little on nutrition, lots on pharmaceutical drugs, and nothing about the effects of processing fats and oils on human health.

—Udo Erasmus

We have been chewing on metaphorical beef jerky this week; it is thick stuff. The topic of dietary fat and its relationship to body fat has been so skewed since the modern processing of fats and oils that this may be all new information to you. You now know that balancing omega-3s and omega-6s is crucial in reducing chronic and acute inflammation, improving your immune system, and sharpening your brain. This week was fat with information! Here is the review:

- Replace your processed fats and oils with the unprocessed varieties and your health will reap the benefits.
- Consuming too much sugar without burning it off results in high triglycerides.
- Remember, every meal and snack should include a healthy fat. As much as 30-50 percent of your daily calories may come from fat. Look back at all prior weeks in this book. Every healthy meal and snack idea includes healthy fat.
- Take small steps. Switch your fat-free dairy to 1 percent or more and exchange your margarine for organic butter. Include healthy fats and extra-virgin oil on your salads and stir-fries or commit to eating wild-caught fish one to two times per week. Pick one food swap and make it a habit!

The Benefits of Healthy Dietary Fat Intake

- Helps you properly absorb fat-soluble vitamins and minerals
- Nourishes your brain
- Protects your nerves
- Keeps you satiated (feeling full) and from overeating
- Aids in proper digestion
- Slows and reverses degenerative diseases
- Levels cholesterol and blood pressure
- Maintains healthy body weight (aka healthy dietary fat does not make you fat)

What Are the Dangers of Not Getting Enough Healthy Dietary Fat?

- Damage to nerves
- Neurological problems (seizures in extreme cases)
- Problems with digestion and irregularity (bowel movements)
- Malnourishment of every cell in the body
- Feeling hungry all day long
- Chronic inflammation
- Low cholesterol
- High blood pressure
- Exacerbation of degenerative diseases

Fats and Oils Can Be Damaged from:

1. Some extraction methods using high heat and/or chemical toxins
2. Adding hydrogen (partially hydrogenated oil)
3. High-heat cooking with delicate oils

Balance Your Omega-3s and -6s

- Eat one to two servings of wild-caught fish per week.
- Add a serving of flaxseed oil or walnuts to your meals or snacks three to four times per week.
- Eat vegetables like winter squash, broccoli, spinach, and cauliflower three to four times per week.
- Limit your foods containing corn and soy products to one or two servings per week *or less*. Always look for non-GMO soy and corn that has been minimally processed.

Recap Questions

Did you make any changes in your fat consumption this week as a result of what you learned? Yes / No? If yes, what changes were made?

_____

_____

_____

_____

This week we learned about dietary fats. We also implemented the sugar challenge. What did you learn from the sugar challenge?

_____

_____

_____

_____

What changes in your sugar consumption do you plan to make this week as a result of the sugar challenge?

_____

_____

_____

_____

How does your consumption affect your relationship with God?

_____

_____

_____

_____

Reflection Notes:

_____

_____

_____

_____

_____

_____

_____

_____

_____

_____

_____

_____

_____

_____

_____

_____

_____

_____

_____

_____

_____

_____

_____

_____

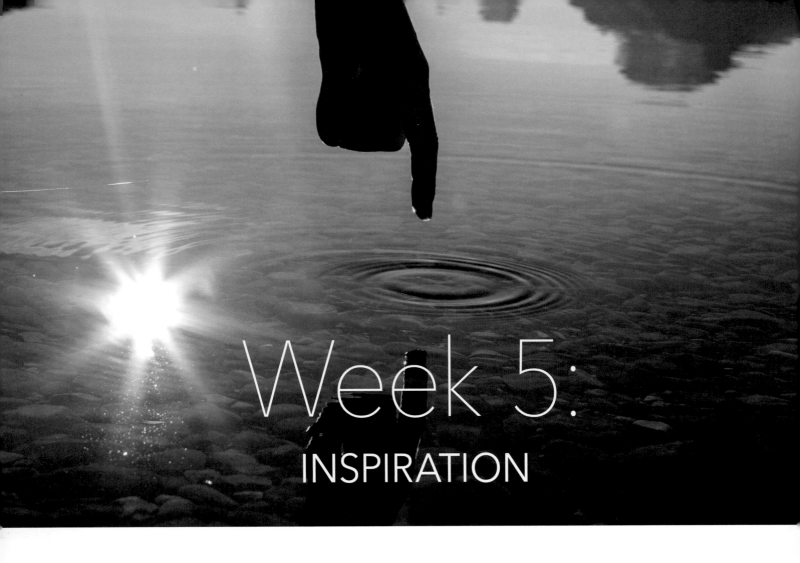

Week 5:
INSPIRATION

Welcome to week 5!

A small drop of water can be seen through its ripple on the other side of the ocean. We consistently become inspired when we acquire the knowledge, become accountable to one another, become more mindful about our decisions, and understand our motivations for our actions. Be inspired to make lasting changes in your health by igniting your intentions into action, and stepping into the person God created you to be.

Inspiration, *noun* in·spi·ra·tion

"Something that makes someone want to do something or that gives someone an idea about what to do or create: a force or influence that inspires someone"

- Source: *Merriam-Webster's Learner's Dictionary*

Week 5 Action Steps

Number one health goal: _____ *Goal Accomplished!* ❑

Accountability

Record your **strength** workouts in the *Living Wellness Journal*;

weekly goal:_____ _____ (number of days) (minutes per day) ❑

    Partner's goal: _____ _____ (number of days) (minutes per day)

Record your **cardio** workouts in the *Living Wellness Journal*;

weekly goal:_____ _____ (number of days) (minutes per day) ❑

    Partner's goal: _____ _____ ❑

What is your **nutrition** goal this week (remember the SMART goals)? _____

_____ ❑ ❑ ❑ ❑ ❑ ❑ ❑

    Partner's nutrition goal: _____ ❑

Record your **food/beverage** intake in *Living Wellness Journal* or app ❑

Check in with your partner daily. ❑ ❑ ❑ ❑ ❑ ❑ ❑

Knowledge

Fill out all questions in this book *prior* to the next meeting. ❑

Mindfulness

Identify your preventable and non-preventable risk factors for osteoporosis (week 5, day 3):

Inspiration

How does the knowledge that God cares about your health inspire your choices?

_____

Motivation

Look back at week 2's motivation action step. Why did you begin this journey? What is your motivation to finish well? _____ ❑

Living Wellness Week 5 Exercise

This week we will be preparing for the grocery store tour. Use this week to do all past exercises!

Looking Ahead

You are over halfway through this part of your journey. This week we will continue to explore our bodies, blood, and bone health. Then we'll end up in the grocery store for inspiration on how to best nourish our bodies!

Week 5, Day 2: Blood Health

Eating adequate fiber is like taking a toothbrush to your digestive system and blood!

There's something special about blood. Blood is precious and life giving. Thinking about blood used to make me squirm a little, and seeing it brought me close to passing out (it still does). But something changed as I began to study and understand the inner workings of the body, and I'm really amazed at the precious and powerful qualities of our blood! Have you thought recently about what your blood does for you?

Blood transports nutrients, cleans cells, and delivers oxygen to the rest of your body.

Why should we care about the health of our blood? *The health of our blood is a key factor to disease prevention!*

How can we care for the health of our blood?

Fiber

Fiber cleans your blood and intestines! Dietary fiber, also known as roughage or bulk, includes all parts of plant foods that your body does not digest or absorb. Fiber acts like magnets and street sweepers moving through your blood and digestive tract. While protein, carbs, and fat break down and absorb in your body, fiber stays intact, attracting toxins that need to be eliminated from your body. Your intestinal tract is about twenty-five feet long—you need all the help you can get to keep that baby clean!

More Benefits of Fiber:

- Balances cholesterol
- Lowers blood sugar levels
- Slows down digestion from the stomach to intestines, increasing nutrient absorption
- Gathers toxins and eliminates them through the digestive system
- Regulates bowel movements
- Helps keep your weight in check by keeping you full after meals and snacks

A 300-calorie meal with 8 grams of fiber will keep you feeling full much longer than a 300-calorie meal with no fiber!

Magnets & Street Sweepers

Soluble Fiber (Magnets)

Soluble fiber acts like a magnet, attracting sugar and toxins to itself. This type of fiber is responsible for balancing cholesterol and blood sugar levels. Soluble fiber is found in, but not limited to, the following:

- Apples
- Legumes
- Citrus fruits
- Peas
- Barley
- Carrots
- Oats
- Psyllium (usually found in fiber supplements)

Insoluble Fiber (Street Sweepers)

Insoluble fiber acts like a street sweeper, gathering the magnets which increase stool bulk and promote the movement of material through your digestive system. It also helps you feel full after meals and snacks. This type of fiber benefits individuals who struggle with constipation or irregular stools. Insoluble fiber is found in but not limited to these foods:

- Legumes
- Green beans
- Potatoes
- 100 percent whole-wheat flour
- Cauliflower
- Nuts
- Wheat bran

As you can see, both soluble and insoluble fiber are needed to ensure your digestive system keeps moving and stays clean. Instead of relying on fiber bars and shakes, which are usually loaded with added sugar, processed oils, and preservatives, most of your fiber should be from raw and steamed veggies, raw fruits, whole grains, and beans. *Consuming a variety of sources offers an important balance of soluble and insoluble fiber.*

How Much Fiber Do You Need?

Mayo Clinic Recommendation:

	Age 50 or younger	Age 51 or older
Men	38 grams	30 grams
Women	25 grams	21 grams

So how much fiber do *you* need per day? _____ grams

Count your servings of fiber for one day and record it here: _____ grams of fiber

Fiber-Rich Foods

- Vegetables (a minimum of two to four servings per day is recommended)

- Fruits (a minimum of one to three servings per day is recommended)

- 100 percent whole grains (zero to three servings per day is recommended—soaked when possible)

- Legumes (one serving per day of either lentils or beans)

We will get plenty of fiber when we consume the recommended amount of each of the above categories. Yet, I often hear that eating healthily is too expensive. How much do fiber supplements cost? How much do diet programs cost? How much do doctor visits cost for digestive problems, chronic illnesses, and preventable diseases? I have struggled with irregular intestinal movements in the past, but it is so refreshing to know that I can be in control of my body. So can you. You make choices every day that affect your health. Make decisions for better health, the raw and organic way.

Do You Need a Fiber Supplement?

Instead of grabbing a fiber bar or shake, try combining:

1 cup blueberries, 3.6 grams fiber

¼ cup walnuts, 1.25 grams fiber

1 tablespoon natural, dark chocolate chips, 1.25 grams fiber

Total Fiber: 6.1 grams (almost 25 percent of your daily fiber needs in one tasty snack!)

That little treat combination is packed with fiber, antioxidants, and healthy fat. Perfect for an energy boost and digestive aid!

If you are still constipated after consuming the recommended fruits, veggies, and beans, there are a few other avenues to explore before you take a fiber supplement—not because they are necessarily bad, but because you may be missing the root cause of the problem.

Constipation Troubleshooting

Are you still constipated? Refer to the Bristol Stool Chart in Appendix E. Remember, any number outside of a number 3 or 4 indicates that there is something wrong in the digestive system.

Do you take medication? If you are eating the recommended fruits, vegetables, and fiber per day and are still constipated, check your medication symptoms and side effects. Some medications cause constipation. Ask your doctor for the most natural remedies available.

- Try more raw fruits and vegetables—Leave the skin on when appropriate and take the time to chew your food (try lightly cooked if you have a hard time digesting raw veggies).

- Water—Are you still drinking half of your ideal body weight in ounces of water? If not, start now. Remember, soluble fiber needs water, to absorb and eliminate toxins from your body.

- Healthy fat—Consuming healthy dietary fats aids in digestion. Try adding one tablespoon of extra-virgin olive oil to your salad and another to your steamed vegetables every day for improved regularity.

- Move more—Your digestive system needs to be exercised just as much as your heart and muscles. Exercise will help the intestines get the bowels moving, from the inside out.

If none of the troubleshooting ideas work and you still want a fiber supplement, look for one with the least amount of additives and sugar. A nutrition response-testing physician may help find an unresolved problem with your digestion.

Too Much of a Good Thing?

You'll always know when you've gotten too much fiber because your body will tell you! Getting too much fiber has adverse effects, such as loose stools, abdominal discomfort, gas, bloating, and intestinal blockage. Such fibers as guar gum, inulin, oligofructose, polydextrose, psyllium, and starch, which are usually found in fiber supplements, have been found to cause abdominal cramping, bloating, gas, and diarrhea—especially when taken in excess.

Also, remember that fiber acts like a magnet for toxins. Too much fiber also acts like a magnet to such minerals as iron, zinc, calcium, and magnesium and can decrease their absorption in your digestive tract. We need those nutrients! Let's not work against our bodies by getting too much of a good thing.

Just the Right Amount

Usually when you begin eliminating ingredients like added sugar, processed carbs, and trans fats from your diet and replacing them with healthy produce, protein, and fat, you lose several pounds within the first week due to elimination. Think about how much food you consume in a day, a week, or a month. If you simply consume less or digest your food with more efficiency, you will lighten up instantly. Eating the right amount of fiber from whole foods assists in your healthy weight and keeps your body detoxified without the need for expensive and complicated cleanses. Natural fiber saves you money!

Take an honest look at what you eat all day. Do you naturally avoid vegetables, beans, lentils, and raw nuts (foods that are high in fiber)? Yes/No

Why?

_____

_____

_____

_____

_____

How will you incorporate more natural sources of fiber into your daily menu?

_____

_____

_____

_____

_____

Fiber cleanses us internally. We also need our external environment to be clean. How can you change your environment to improve your relationship with God? (i.e. music, friends, habits, books, media, exercise). Read more in Romans 12: 1-2 and James 4:7-8

_____

_____

_____

_____

_____

_____

Week 5, Day 3: Bone and Joint Health

Let food be thy medicine and medicine be thy food.

—Hippocrates

If you're a young person who thinks you can skip this reading, think again. How you treat your body today will directly impact the diseases you will or won't fight tomorrow, including osteoporosis and arthritis!

As we age, we often think that breaking bones and wearing cartilage is just a normal part of growing old. The reality is that we do not have to lose all our bone density and soft tissue, but it takes intentional action to keep our muscles and bones strong and healthy.

Osteoporosis is a result of bone loss and/or the body ceasing to make bone tissue. The National Osteoporosis Foundation (NOF) states: "About 10 million Americans have osteoporosis. About 34 million are at risk for the disease. Estimates suggest that about half of all women older than 50, and up to one in four men, will break a bone because of osteoporosis."

Osteoarthritis is a similar condition that results from worn-down cartilage that covers the ends of bones at a joint. Osteoarthritis causes joint pain and reduced range of motion.

Osteoporosis and osteoarthritis affect both men and women, but women are more at risk for the diseases. The conditions are more common in mature adults. They are expensive and debilitating diseases. *Osteoporosis and osteoarthritis are not inevitable with aging.* We can protect our bones and soft tissue at all stages of life. According to the NOF, there are uncontrollable and controllable risk factors that should be considered with osteoporosis.

Uncontrollable Risk Factors (NOF)

- Being over age fifty
- Being female
- Menopause
- Family history
- Past broken bones or height loss

Controllable Risk Factors (NOF)

- Not getting enough calcium and vitamin D
- Not eating enough fruits and vegetables
- Getting too much sodium and caffeine
- Having an inactive lifestyle

- Smoking
- Drinking too much alcohol
- Being overweight

Below are the four main ways to prevent and lessen the symptoms of osteoporosis and osteoarthritis:

1. Balanced nutrition

2. Resistance or strength training

3. Avoiding smoking

4. Limiting alcohol

What are your uncontrollable risk factors?

_____

_____

_____

_____

_____

_____

What are your controllable risk factors?

_____

_____

_____

_____

_____

_____

Week 5, Day 4:
Balancing Calcium and Vitamin D for Bone Health

My solid body and strong bones are a result of my nutrition and physical activity growing up on a dairy farm. Fresh, organic whole milk and my daily physical lifestyle laid the foundation for my strong body. Now I keep myself healthy by limiting sugar, eating plenty of fruits and vegetables, and exercising my body as often as I can. —Donna S., inFIT client

We all know that calcium is good for maintaining strong bones. The 2010 recommendation from the National Academy of Sciences is that people ages nineteen to fifty consume 1,000 milligrams of calcium per day and that those age fifty or over get 1,200 milligrams per day.

It takes a variety of only two to three servings of dairy, almond milk, or coconut milk per day to reach 1,200 milligrams per day. You can also incorporate a variety of vegetables, fruits, nuts, and seeds to make up the difference.

Good Sources of Calcium

- 2 tablespoons blackstrap molasses, 400 mg of calcium
- 1 cup collards, bok choy, and baked beans, approximately 350 mg of calcium
- Natural supplements that contain both calcium and vitamin D3, ranges from 300-1,000 mg of calcium
- 1 cup organic raw milk, plain yogurt, cheese, eggs, and other organic, pasture-raised sources of dairy, approximately 300-500 mg of calcium
- 1 cup unsweetened almond milk, approximately 100 mg of calcium
- 1 tablespoon sesame seeds, 88 mg of calcium
- 1 ounce of nuts like almonds and Brazil nuts, approximately 75 mg of calcium
- 1 large orange, 74 mg of calcium
- 1 cup unsweetened almonds, approximately 38 mg of calcium
- 1 cup vegetables like spinach, kelp, broccoli, and celery, approximately 30 mg of calcium

Too Much of a Good Thing?

What most people do not know is that too much calcium, by itself, can be harmful. The Mayo Clinic states that "too much calcium has risks." Research indicates that too much calcium (an excess of 1,200 milligrams in women and 2,000 milligrams in men) has been linked with ovarian and prostate cancers. It is important to consume calcium from a wide variety of sources, and it is best to combine it with foods containing vitamin D and magnesium for optimal absorption.

Vitamin D

Calcium without vitamin D decreases the calcium absorption in your body. In addition to maintaining strong bones, vitamin D also has these benefits:

- Prevents autoimmune diseases
- Prevents several types of cancers
- Reduces the risk of cardiovascular disease

How Much Vitamin D Do You Need?

Women and Men	
Under age 50	**Age 50 and older**
400-800 international units (IU) daily*	800–1,000 IU daily*

*Some individuals need more vitamin D than others. According to the Institute of Medicine (IOM), the safe upper limit of vitamin D is 4,000 IU per day for most adults. Check with your doctor if you think you need more vitamin D.

Sources of Vitamin D

There are three ways to get vitamin D:

1. Food

2. Sunlight

3. Supplements (be sure the labels list Vitamin D3, which is a much more absorbable form than Vitamin D2)

What Is "Fortified"?

Dairy products are often labeled "fortified" with vitamin D to make them more attractive. "Fortified" means that supplements have been added to a food or beverage. If your food is fortified with the natural Vitamin D3, enjoy in moderation! However, in most cases, to reduce manufacturing costs, foods are fortified with synthetic vitamins. Read ingredient labels.

What Are Synthetic Vitamins?

Synthetic vitamins and supplements are created in a lab to look and feel like natural vitamins and minerals, however they are anything but natural. Synthetic vitamins and minerals have a negative impact on our health. Several organizations (below) have researched the effects of synthetic or fortified nutrients on our bodies. Some of the side effects include:

- Interfering with the absorption of nutrients (Organic Consumers Association)
- Causing fat-soluble vitamins to build up in unhealthy levels (Organic Consumers Association)
- Causing birth defects (1995 *New England Journal of Medicine* study)
- Causing blood clotting (Dr. Maret Traber, professor of nutrition at the Linus Pauling Institute)
- Causing hypercalcemia—buildup of calcium in the blood (National Institutes of Health)
- Increasing risk of cancer (*Journal of the National Cancer Institute*, 2004)

Buying a generic, synthetic multivitamin is not going to ensure balanced calcium and vitamin D. If you think you need a supplement, first check with your doctor or a doctor who performs nutrition response testing to see what you need. Then find organic supplements from a quality source rather than a synthetic variety.

Foods Containing Vitamin D

Sushi (raw fish)—Sushi contains higher levels of vitamin D than cooked fish, but do not force yourself if you do not like raw fish; cooked varieties still offer ample amounts of the nutrient. Keep in mind that sushi rolls usually contain very little raw fish but have an overabundance of white rice, a processed carbohydrate that will fill you up without the nourishment, leading to an increase in sugar cravings. When in doubt, go without (white rice, that is). Or, if you have the option, ask for your sushi roll to be made with brown rice.

Fish—Canned and fresh salmon, canned and fresh mackerel, oil-packed sardines, and oil-packed tuna provide around half of the recommended daily value of vitamin D. Fish is great with vegetables, on salads, or served from the grill.

Oysters—Yes, I cringe at this one, but if you like oysters, good news—keep eating them in moderation! In addition to the 80 percent of your daily value in vitamin D, oysters provide a great source of copper, iron, manganese, selenium, vitamin B12, and zinc.

Caviar (black and red)—Served on whole-grain crackers or fish, caviar provides around 50 percent of your daily need for vitamin D per teaspoon.

Dairy products—Most dairy products, such as milk and cheese, contains small amounts of vitamin D. Raw is best, but if raw dairy is not available, always buy dairy from organic, grass-fed animals to avoid exposure to harmful chemicals. Organic dairy does cost more, but you can balance the added cost by consuming less dairy.

Organic eggs and mushrooms—these foods offer a relatively low amount of vitamin D, but combined with other foods, they can be an easy and delicious way to get 100 percent of your daily intake!

Vitamin D supplements*—Taking a vitamin D supplement may be an important avenue if you are not getting enough of the nutrient from food or sunlight. Investigate the consumer reports, find a naturopath, or ask a physician (who has nutrition training) to discover which supplements are receiving high-quality ratings. Remember, Vitamin D3 is what you should be looking for on the label.

*Individuals with elevated serum calcium levels or hyperparathyroidism should not take vitamin D without consulting a physician.

Why did I leave out soy from this list? Soy does include vitamin D, but soy also acts like estrogen in your body. According to the National Institute of Environmental Health Sciences (NIEHS), too much estrogen in the body is directly linked with several types of cancer. For instance, if you have a thyroid imbalance, it may be beneficial to avoid soy products. If your soy comes from the United States, it is probably genetically modified (GMO or GM) unless otherwise specified. Watch out for soy in things that you may not think of like chocolate, chewing gum, chips, and processed foods. Be cautious of consuming too many soy products.

Sunlight

As previously stated, your body produces vitamin D when it comes in contact with sunlight, specifically the UVB rays. Getting short but regular exposure to sunlight can be a great (and refreshing) way to keep your bones strong and healthy. And did you know that by eating citrus fruits or adding fresh lemon to your water, you get an antioxidant boost that protects against sun damage? Eat your fruits and vegetables when you are out in the sun!

If you are concerned about skin cancer, limit your direct sun exposure to ten minutes or less *and* get a variety of vitamin D through food and supplementation. Talk to your physician about what the best option is for you.

Too Much of a Good Nutrient?

As with any nutrient, stay within your recommended amounts. Too much vitamin D can put you at risk for kidney damage.

Of the list of vitamin D-rich foods, which will you commit to consume on a regular basis?

_____

_____

Week 5, Day 5: Resistance Training for Strong Bones

How is resistance training different from cardiovascular training? Why is it relevant to weight loss and bone density?

1. According to the Harvard School of Public Health, "Strength training, also known as resistance training, weight training, or muscle-strengthening activity, is probably the most neglected component of fitness programs but one of the most beneficial."

2. Cardio training is meant to work your heart, whereas strength training is designed to improve your muscle tone and bone mineral density.

How Does Strength Training Increase Bone Mineral Density?

Bearing weight on the muscles and bones causes them to react to the stressors. The increase in your muscle seems obvious—work your muscles and they get stronger. Your bones react the same way. Put consistent, appropriate resistance on your bones and they get stronger!

Think about a tree that grows up solely in a greenhouse, sheltered from all external environments. If left inside its whole life, the tree usually matures with small roots and a weak trunk. Without proper nutrients, sunshine, and natural elements, such as wind and temperature, it never experiences the opportunity to fully develop. Once the fragile adult tree is put outside in the wind, rain, and variable temperature, it snaps and breaks. However, if that tree is nourished and periodically taken out of the greenhouse to experience elements like wind and rain, it will grow thicker, tougher, and be able to handle the natural environment. Our bodies are similar to the trees. When we avoid resistance training and malnourish our bodies, we are at risk to bend and snap like trees sheltered from natural challenges.

On the other hand, if we nourish and condition our muscles and bones to handle resistance training, they become stronger and abler to handle physical stress. In addition to increasing bone mineral density, full-body strength training has a multitude of benefits, including:

- Reduced back pain
- Reduced stress
- Increased balance
- Improved sleep
- Reduced risk of injury
- Improved blood flow
- Improved circulation
- Improved self-image
- Increased metabolism

If you haven't already, get a bone density test and a noninvasive muscle percentage test from a doctor and a professionally certified trainer as you start or continue strength training. Once you begin your strength routine

It's never too late to be more fit!

(I hope that you've been practicing the strength workouts in this book), watch your muscle percentage and bone density increase. It's never too late to be more fit!

No Excuses Needed

Are you stuck in a chair from bad knees? Work your upper body and core.

Are you still hurting from an old shoulder injury? Work your lower body and core.

If you can move your body, you can strengthen your body. Recruit the help of a professional if you do not know how to start.

Are you currently doing strength training? If not, when do you plan to start, specifically?

_____

_____

_____

How Much Resistance Training Should You Do Each Week?

To improve your current physical condition, add two to three hours of strength training per week. Unless you split the workout by muscle group, the Living Wellness Workouts provided in this book may be performed no more than two to three times per week, as they are full-body resistance training workouts (and you need at least forty-eight hours of rest between strength sessions on the same muscle groups).

If you aren't currently strength training, it's not too late to start! Almost everyone can add strength training to his or her routine. The benefits far outweigh the postexercise muscle burn.

The number-one thing that keeps me motivated to take care of myself is my three beautiful girls. We all need exercise, sleep, and healthy foods to be the best we can be at whatever we are doing—I want to model these behaviors so that my girls have the knowledge and confidence to make healthy choices for the rest of their lives!

—Jill Mischke, certified personal trainer

Week 5, Day 6: Vitamins and Supplements

In his book *The Most Effective Natural Cures on Earth*, Jonny Bowden, PhD, assembles his list of desert island cures with foods and supplements. Through the course of my journey, and with the help of naturopaths, I have I assembled a list of my own "Desert Island Cures," which include magnesium, garlic, mineral salt, apple cider vinegar, probiotics, and fish oil. Remember, there are no cure-alls, but some foods do have a more powerful healing effect than others. And, as we are all different, our bodies have different needs in regard to nutrition and supplementation. As you listen and respond to *your* body's needs, you will discover a balance that keeps you well. We will examine apple cider vinegar and probiotics later, so now let's examine magnesium.

Magnesium

Magnesium is one of those notably necessary but often neglected nutrients in our diet. Bowden suggests magnesium as one of his "Desert Island Cures," pointing out that one out of four Americans do not get the recommended daily value. Magnesium affects every cell in your body; it affects your metabolism and energy production. Not getting enough magnesium can result in any of the following problems:

- Salt and sugar cravings
- Cramps
- Insomnia
- Muscle tensions
- Poor blood sugar control
- Worsened allergy symptoms

- Cardiovascular disease
- Increased premenstrual symptoms
- Mitral valve prolapse
- Panic attacks
- Weakened immune system

This is quite a list for a rather "unknown" mineral. However, I've seen the transformation in several people, including my husband and me, with allergies, cravings, and PMS (the latter is more for me, but you know that affects him too).

Garlic

Allicin is the powerful antioxidant within garlic that helps your body maintain balanced levels of cholesterol and a healthy heart. Garlic has been used for centuries as a remedy for heart health and the treatment of common illnesses. In a study dated January 2009, in an issue of the *International Journal of Chemistry*, Angewandte Chemie confirms this folk remedy, describing garlic as one of the most powerful antioxidants available. Antioxidants are responsible for fighting free radicals, reversing signs of aging, and killing bacteria in your body. Add a clove to your veggies, salad, or chicken breast to fight free radicals in your body instantly. The less you cook garlic, the higher the antioxidant value will be. If you don't love the flavor of fresh garlic, try lightly steaming it with your veggies to begin to train your palate!

Why Is Mineral Salt Important?

Mineral salt is important because it contains a variety of minerals, including sodium. Sodium is an essential mineral that is also found in some vegetables and seafood. Sodium plays an important role in the regulation of your body's electrical and nerve functions. Sodium also plays a vital role in regulating nutrients in and out of every cell in your body and regulating your blood pressure. Because of the phrase *heart disease*, we as a nation are afraid of salt. Many people avoid sodium because of its link to heart disease. The problem is not sodium. The problem is either too much sodium from processed salt (sodium chloride) or not enough sodium because we are afraid of it.

When we do not get enough sodium, the result is hyponatremia, a metabolic condition in which salt and water are dangerously out of balance between the inside and outside of our cells.

One of my colleagues passed out at my fitness center a while back. His trauma was one of the scariest things I have been through. He was teaching a class when he felt off balance. He went to the bathroom to try to regain control of his shaky body, and he fainted. We called for an ambulance as he remained unconscious. He was brought to the hospital for a battery of tests for his heart, lungs, and brain. After checking all his body's vitals, blood counts, and minerals, the symptoms suggested hyponatremia. Hyponatremia can be life threatening and may cause brain herniation, possible coma, or even death.

I do not point this out to scare you. Rather, I want you to take great care in getting enough and the right kind of salt in your diet. Let's review one of the S's of the FOSS chart.

FOSS	Processed Food (Toxic)–Avoid	Less Processed (Some Health Benefits)	Unprocessed (Nourishing)– Enjoy in Moderation	Enjoy with Reckless Abandon
Salt	Table salt, sodium nitrite, sodium nitrate Monosodium glutamate (MSG)	Kosher salt Commercial sea salt	Unrefined mineral salt, such as Celtic sea salt or pink Himalayan (generally, salt should have a color)	MODERATION

Remember to read labels to avoid processed salt in packaged foods.

As you change your habits from eating processed and packaged foods to whole foods, I encourage you to experiment with different kinds of mineral salts. Throw away the sodium chloride (table salt) from the pantry and get out the salt grinder! Your taste buds will be excited to try the different flavors found in real mineral salt.

How Much Sodium Do We Need?

"The 2010 Dietary Guidelines for Americans recommends limiting sodium to less than 2,300 milligrams a day—or 1,500 milligrams if you are age fifty-one or older, if you are black, or if you have high blood pressure, diabetes, or chronic kidney disease," according to the Mayo Clinic.

Take notice of how much and the type of sodium you consume on a regular basis. Getting enough but not overdoing sodium is an essential part of feeling good, protecting your heart, and stepping off of the "sick and tired" roller coaster.

What Are the Best Sources of Sodium?

- Vegetables! Artichokes, beets, carrots, seaweed, turnips, beet greens, celery, and chard contain 75 milligrams of sodium or more per serving. When cooked without salt, sweet potatoes, spinach, and collards contain 75 milligrams of sodium or more per serving.
- All mineral salts, but especially salts high in trace minerals, such as:
  - Celtic sea salt (especially for low thyroid functioning conditions)
  - Pink Himalayan salt (Think: most of the time, real salt has a color!)
- Seafood
- Cheese

Iodine in Salt

Iodine is an essential nutrient for your body. Iodine is marketed on some table salt as a great "source" of the nutrient. However, the iodine found in most table salt (sodium chloride) is synthetic, and although we might be fooled, our bodies are not.

Consuming synthetic iodine usually results in an iodine deficiency and a potentially under-functioning thyroid due to constant exposure to elements that cause an imbalance in your body's essential nutrients. Most manufacturers are looking for the cheapest way to mass-produce foods and condiments we use every day.

Obtain iodine naturally from such foods as mineral salt, kale, egg yolk, tuna, garlic, asparagus, and spinach rather than from fortified table salt. Whole foods are nourishing and give your body the balance of minerals it is looking for.

If you think you are low in any vitamins or minerals, check with your naturopath, nutrition response tester, or doctor to see if adding one or more may be beneficial to help manage your weight, manage your cravings, and get you off the roller coaster of "sick and tired."

What kind of salt are you using? Are you open to switching to a natural mineral salt?

_____

_____

_____

_____

How would you benefit from visiting a naturopath or nutrition response tester?

_____

_____

_____

_____

_____

_____

_____

_____

_____

_____

_____

_____

_____

_____

_____

_____

Week 5, Day 7: Recap & Reflect

Balanced Body, Balanced Mind

Your blood is amazing. Take care of your blood by eating plenty of natural fiber (vegetables and beans) and exercising on a regular basis. Another way to keep your blood healthy (that isn't covered in this book) is to reduce the exposure to chemicals from your skin care and home cleaning products. There are plenty of publications you can read if you want to reduce your exposure to environmental toxins. Check Appendix H for my book lists by subject. For now, let's recap the week:

- The benefits of fiber include balancing cholesterol, lowering blood sugar levels, gathering toxins and eliminating them through the digestive system, regulating bowel movements, and helping keep your weight in check by keeping you full after meals and snacks

- Eat fiber naturally from a variety of vegetables, legumes, nuts, and fruits. Avoid fiber supplements.

- Your bones and joints *need to move* in order to be strong and healthy! You also need to nourish your body in order to support the health of your bones and joints. Getting enough natural vitamin D, calcium, fruit, and vegetables is a promising start to support the structure that's going to support you—for life!

Eating well on every budget starts with good planning. This does not have to be intensive. Purchase nonperishables in bulk and prepare several meals at a time to save money (and the need for fast food). Learn how to use a whole chicken rather than just buying the breasts or thighs.

- Supplementation is a billion-dollar industry because most people want to live longer and feel better. We want to lose weight and look younger. Avoid the trap of taking supplements without a purpose.

- Supplementation is really individual, based on the needs of your body. My best advice for your bio-individual supplementation is to find a holistic nutritionist, a doctor who offers nutrition response testing, or a naturopath who is recommended and trusted. Get tested to find out specifically what your body needs during various seasons, what nutrients it absorbs well, and what it does not. Until you receive an individual supplementation plan, make sure your body's most essential nutrients are balanced. Remember, health is a way of life; health is *not* dependent on the next miracle cure.

- Muscle burns body fat. Strength training allows your body to burn fat when you are sitting at a desk, watching a movie, or even sleeping! Strength training has benefits beyond strong bones.

Reflection Questions

How do you plan on consuming more natural fiber this week?

_____

_____

_____

What new strength training exercise will you try this week?

_____

_____

_____

Have you experienced less anxiety and more brain clarity when you nourish your body?
Please explain.

_____

_____

_____

How do you nourish your mind, body, and spirit before walking into stressful situations?

_____

_____

_____

Reflection Notes:

_____

_____

_____

_____

_____

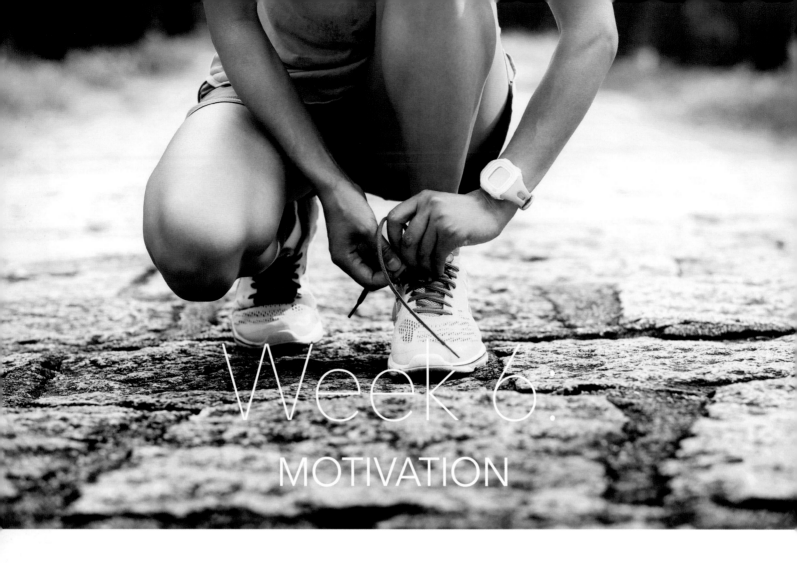

Week 6:
MOTIVATION

Welcome to week 6!

Remember back to week 1 when we talked about your root why? We will continue thinking about your "why" for health. Hopefully you have been thinking about *why* you desire to be healthier these past six weeks. Thinking about your motives and being mindful with your decisions will make a positive difference in your long-term success and in the journey along the way! Why does God want you to be well and whole?

**The thief comes only to steal and kill
and destroy. I came that they may have life
and have it abundantly.**

- John 10:10 (ESV)

Today in the Living Wellness Growth Group, we'll be going to the grocery store to bring the FOSS Chart to life! If you're working through this study on your own, commit to getting to the grocery store this week to practice an in-depth look at labels, using the FOSS Chart as your guide.

Week 6 Action Steps

Number one health goal: _____ *Goal Accomplished!* ❏

Accountability

Record your **strength** workouts in the *Living Wellness Journal*;

weekly goal:_____ _____ (number of days) (minutes per day) ❏

       Partner's goal: _____ _____ (number of days) (minutes per day)

Record your **cardio** workouts in the *Living Wellness Journal*;

weekly goal:_____ _____ (number of days) (minutes per day) ❏

       Partner's goal: _____ _____ ❏

What is your **nutrition** goal this week (remember the SMART goals)? _____

_____ ❏ ❏ ❏ ❏ ❏ ❏

       Partner's nutrition goal: _____ ❏

Record your **food/beverage** intake in *Living Wellness Journal* or app ❏

Check in with your partner daily. ❏ ❏ ❏ ❏ ❏ ❏

Knowledge

Fill out all questions in this book *prior* to the next meeting. ❏ ❏ ❏ ❏ ❏ ❏ ❏

Mindfulness

Practice making your own fermented food this week (see shopping list below). ❏

Inspiration

Next time you go grocery shopping, ask God to give you wisdom and guidance. ❏

Motivation

What is one thing you can do this week to better manage your stress? _____ ❏

Living Wellness Week 6 Exercises

Add these two exercises to your existing strength training routine.

Reverse Fly

With a neutral spine, hinge forward until your back is at about a 45-degree angle. Keep your core tight and inhale as you drop your hands directly below your shoulders, rounding out your elbows. Exhale as you lift your hands up to be in line with your shoulders. Your elbows should still be slightly bent.

For Option II, perform reverse fly in a split stance (lunge position).

Perform 16 to 20 reps or for the single-arm rows, 8 to 10 reps on each leg. Repeat as time permits.

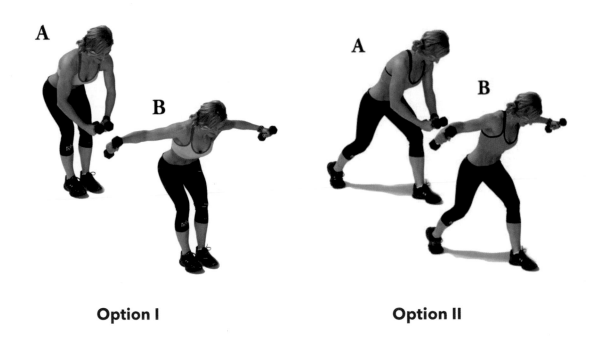

Option I   **Option II**

Bridges

Lie on your back and bend your knees. Your feet should be about six inches from your butt. Inhale as you pull your belly button into your spine and flatten your low back against the ground. Exhale as you lift your hips off the ground. You should lift your hips so that they are in line with your shoulders and knees, no higher. Tighten your butt muscles.

For Option II, lift one leg straight in the air and lift your hips.

Perform 16 to 20 reps or 8 to 10 on each leg. Repeat as time permits. Do these exercises every other day. Remember to stretch after your workout.

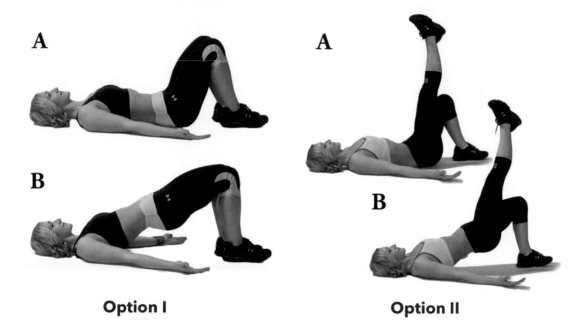

Option I   **Option II**

Looking Ahead

This week, we will explore one of the most mysterious (and interesting) parts of the body—the gut.

Shopping List for Fermented Foods

This week, you will practice making your own fermented foods! Pick up the ingredients below to make sauerkraut, Sauerkraut Auflauf, and sourdough bread on days 4, 5, and 6, respectively.

Sauerkraut

1 cabbage
2 tablespoons mineral salt (pink Himalayan or Celtic salt are great options)

Sauerkraut Auflauf

½ pound red-skinned potatoes (lower starch levels)
2 tablespoons organic butter
8–16 ounces sauerkraut (you will find the balance you like if you make it a couple of times; I would go for less potatoes than sauerkraut)
One fresh pineapple, or canned in its own juice
16 ounces shredded cheese (I prefer pepper jack)

Sourdough Starter and Bread

Making your own sourdough starter takes five days, so if you want to bake bread on day 5, you need to start your starter today. Refer to day 5 on how to get your starter started today. If you have a starter from a friend, you can keep it in the fridge until you are ready to make bread.

Ingredients for Sourdough Starter

1 bag (at least 8 cups) organic 100 percent whole-wheat flour or organic bread flour (my favorite brand is King Arthur Organic 100% Bread Flour)
4 cups filtered water

WEEK 6

Your grocery list:

_____
_____
_____
_____
_____
_____
_____
_____
_____
_____
_____
_____
_____
_____
_____
_____
_____
_____
_____
_____
_____
_____

MOTIVATION

Week 6, Day 2: The Gut Balance

Talking about gut health is where my personal story returns to the stage.

I used to get sick a lot. Even as a fitness professional, my colleagues would say, "You are the healthiest sick person I know." I blamed my constant illness on bad genes and having children that brought home *the bug*. Sinus infections, common colds, pinkeye (yes, as an adult), strep throat, asthma, allergies, adult acne, influenza, and the stomach flu: I had all of it, all the time. However, I had a gradual awareness that my illnesses were wearing on my family and me. I hit the breaking point of being sick and tired many years ago, and I have rarely looked back.

After trying every cream, pill, and supplement on the market, I went to see a nutrition response tester (Kelley Suggs) for my acne. With a few tests, Kelley determined that my acne and most other illnesses were a direct result of candida, a problem in my gut. I knew that the gut was an important part of digestion, but back then, I didn't know how important the gut was in relation to every other aspect of my health and immunity.

After months of cutting out all sugar and fruit, and eating plenty of gut-healing foods such as bone broth and vegetables, my skin cleared up and my allergies were gone! At first I was skeptical, but when I slipped back into old habits and my symptoms returned, I knew that I did indeed have gut issues that needed to be dealt with once and for all.

It took another wellness expert to help me discover that we need each other in this journey. We have blind spots and stubborn habits. Our friends help us remember our priorities and make choices based on them. I went in to see Kelley for my acne; I left her office with a health transformation.

After my life-changing transformation, I decided to faithfully and consistently live out what I have been teaching for so long. When I stopped getting ill and no longer struggled with my weight and adult acne, I finally understood why I had been always getting sick; the former me thought I was healthy–*for the most part*.

Pause. I just said it: for the most part. Looking back at my sick and overweight years, I am honest with myself (now) that I did not consistently eat enough vegetables, pay attention to balancing healthy fats (remember the immune-boosting effects of omega-3s), drink enough water, eat fermented foods, eat only 100 percent whole grains, consistently take my vitamins, learn to delegate and manage my stress, and avoid sugar like a cavity. I was a *sugar addict*, disguising my issues by being mostly fit and mostly happy with my body. I had moments before my transformation when I hit a personal record for strength gains or even went for a month without getting a cold, but as soon as I treated my gut badly, the pounds accrued and I attracted a stomach bug.

The knowledge of how to take care of my gut has dramatically impacted my family's health and well-being. And now that my gut is healed, I'm able to enjoy fruit and healthy treats in moderation. Life is amazing in our family when Mom is healthy–everyone seems to stay healthy, and when Mom is sick, everyone gets sick (leaving no one to take care of Mom).

Can you relate to the pain of my past struggles? I hope not, but if you do, read on; gut health applies to all of us.

After reading my story, which of your issues do you feel are connected to *your* gut health?

_____

_____

_____

_____

_____

_____

_____

_____

We will examine gut health in detail this week, but let's overview how to get started balancing your gut environment today:

- Avoid excessive sugar intake.
- Drink filtered water.
- Consume gut-healing foods such as bone broth and leafy green vegetables.
- Consume a variety of fermented foods such as pickles and vinegar daily.
- Manage chronic stress with exercise.

How will *you* get started balancing your gut?

_____

_____

_____

_____

_____

_____

_____

_____

Week 6, Day 3: Fermentation and the Gut

Fermentation has been around since ancient times and has been studied extensively since the 1500s with the invention of the compound microscope. Fermentation is the process of adding microorganisms, such as mold, yeast, or bacteria, to foods and beverages to break down or digest compounds and nutrients. Your body does this naturally when you eat; your stomach naturally produces chemicals to break down your food. Yet, often we do not have *enough* natural bacteria (flora, gut bacteria, and probiotics) in our stomach. Also, some foods (grains and proteins) need more assistance than others to break down and digest. Fermented foods and beverages are an integral part of proper digestion.

Examples of fermented foods and beverages include:

- Apple cider vinegar and other vinegars (e.g. rice, wine, and balsamic) *Avoid white distilled vinegar as it's usually made from highly processed corn
- Yogurt, kefir, and some cultured cheese
- Certain breads like sourdough and ciabatta
- Pickled vegetables (sauerkraut, pickles, beets, etc.)
- Wine, beer, and other alcoholic beverages

Most people don't like the taste of sour foods because we don't eat them—but remember, *we crave what we eat*, so if you're not already doing this, eat more fermented foods! Slowly introduce your gut to fermented foods if you're not currently eating them.

Benefits of Consuming a Variety of Fermented Foods Daily

Fermented foods help your body break down and absorb nutrients, boost your immune system, and keep your bowels regular. Fermented foods also support necessary bacteria in your digestive tract. Your body's natural supply of flora gets crushed from certain medications, chlorinated water, and antibiotics in our foods; we need good bacteria on a daily basis to keep the balance of flora in our bodies.

Remember when we compared our metabolism to a flow of traffic? Think of that flow of traffic again and imagine if the cars traveling through the streets and intersections were the food in our bodies, and the necessary bacteria are the stoplights. If you do not have any stoplights (lack of good bacteria from consuming too much chlorine in tap water or antibiotics in meat and dairy), the streets will get congested and backed up with cars (constipation). When there are too many cars in one place for too long, chemicals start to build up (bad bacteria in our stomachs). Car jams and congested roads lead to polluted cities and frustrated people. When we do not properly digest our food, an imbalance of bad bacteria builds up, causing toxicity within the gut.

For example, imagine eating a few slices of pizza knowing they will sit and rot in your gut for a couple of days if they do not digest properly. The undigested food becomes like a magnet for disease-causing bacteria. Where are the stoplights to keep that pizza flowing through your body in a timely manner? A healthy portion of fiber will help move the pizza along, but not until the pizza is broken down will it travel all the way through the digestive tract. Healthy bacteria and fermented foods and beverages will help to digest the pizza so that the fiber you ate can take out the garbage.

If you have ever heard that a six-ounce glass of red wine per day is good for you, the benefits of fermentation support that statement. But, as in all good things, more than what is beneficial means harmful. Limit your consumption of alcoholic beverages and instead focus on consuming a variety of other fermented foods and beverages. If you do not drink alcohol, there is no need to start. Too much alcohol adds calories and a host of other negative side effects, including nerve damage, liver damage, heart damage, brain damage, withdrawal, damage to unborn children, and sexual disorders.

There are many other ways to gradually incorporate fermented foods into your nutrition plan:

- Add organic apple cider vinegar or balsamic vinegar to your salad or steamed veggies.

- Replace your regular bread with a fresh sourdough variety.

- Add plain kefir or yogurt to your smoothies.

- Drink kombucha—a fermented beverage found in grocery and natural food stores. You can also make your own! Instructions are found in Appendix A. Ask around. You may have a friend who is willing to share a SCOBY (symbiotic colony of bacteria and yeast). Your facilitator may have one for purchase or Kombuchakamp.com is another resource to explore.

- Add fermented vegetables like pickled cucumbers, beets, kimchi, onions, salsa, and sauerkraut to meals and snacks. Remember to read labels and compare against the FOSS Chart to avoid unwanted ingredients.

- Add a tablespoon of fermented chutney to cooked poultry or beef.

Practice fermenting your own foods! Have the courage to discover what you like and what you do not.

Of the above list, what fermented food or beverage are you willing to try?

_____

_____

_____

Do you have your groceries to make sauerkraut and sourdough bread this week? Half the battle of cooking is having the right ingredients and making something for the first time.

If it's just not going to be possible to make them from scratch, do the next best thing—buy them pre-made!

Week 6, Day 4: Sauerkraut!

Today, we're going to make sauerkraut! This recipe is so quick and easy and has an unbelievably different flavor than store-bought sauerkraut. Even if you haven't enjoyed sauerkraut in the past, I encourage you to be brave and adventurous and try it homemade. If your recipe doesn't turn out right the first time, try, try again!

Homemade, Small-Batch Sauerkraut Recipe

Ingredients and Tools Needed

1 medium cabbage
1-1 ½ tablespoons mineral salt—non-iodized
Bowl—bigger is better
2-quart wide-mouth canning jar with plastic lid or a wide mouth jar with a metal bale
Shredder or sharp knife
Measuring spoons

Directions

1. Chop the cabbage into fourths and then shred or slice finely. I like to slice mine so there is more crunch and less mush. Put all the sliced or shredded cabbage in a large bowl.

2. Add 1-1 ½ tablespoons of salt to the bowlful of shredded or finely sliced cabbage. Remember to use mineral salt, but make sure it is non-iodized or fermentation won't happen. Now for the magic . . .

3. Wash your hands. Roll up your sleeves and massage the cabbage for up to ten minutes. Water will begin to release from the cabbage. Keep going until the cabbage becomes limp.

4. Pack the cabbage tightly into your jar with your closed fist. Repeat until almost all the cabbage is in the jar, getting it as full as possible. Pour the liquid into the jar.

5. Fill the jar to the top, add water if needed, and seal the lid. The key to making a small batch of sauerkraut is to use a wide-mouth jar with a rubber gasket and wire bale. It's perfect for one head of cabbage. The wire bale allows the liquid to release from the jar during the fermentation process.

6. Place the closed jar in a bowl, as liquid may be released during the first few days. The wire fastener keeps a tight fit while still allowing liquid to escape. Store it in a cool, dark place for 5–10 days. Fermentation takes longer in cold weather and less time in warm climates.

7. Enjoy! Be careful when opening for the first time, as there may be a geyseric effect. I always open mine for the first time in the sink. Store in the refrigerator and enjoy your delicious, probiotic-rich sauerkraut!

Now, you can eat your sauerkraut plain or warmed up with a little melted Swiss cheese, or you can save for day 5 for an all-out authentic German treat.

Week 6, Day 5: Sauerkraut Auflauf Recipe

From the author of the *Living Wellness Devotional*, Christina's famous "Sauerkraut Auflauf" story and recipe follows. Christina is a native German.

In the past, I did not like sauerkraut–I know, that is un-German of me. Leaving Germany, learning more about optimal nutrition, missing my mother's comforting cuisine, and being asked all the time if I eat sauerkraut, I found myself trying to reconstruct my mother's famous sauerkraut dish.

It turns out to be prepared almost in a dash of salt (I love that in a recipe!), and Americans love this dish wherever I have served it!

–Christina Zaczkowski, author of *Living Wellness Devotional*

Ingredients:

½ pound red-skinned potatoes (lower starch levels)
2 tablespoons organic butter
8–16 ounces sauerkraut (you will find the balance you like if you make it a couple of times; I would go for less potatoes than sauerkraut)
One fresh pineapple, or canned in its own juice
16 ounces shredded cheese (I prefer pepper jack)

Instructions:

- Boil (to peel or not to peel, that is your preference!) potatoes until soft to make mashed potatoes with an appropriate amount of organic butter.

- While the potatoes boil, drain one serving of sauerkraut.

- Cut up pineapple or open can and drain the juice (or drink the juice).

- Preheat the oven to 425 degrees Fahrenheit.

- When potatoes are mashed, spread flat on the bottom of a deep-dish pan.

- Spread pineapple chunks over the mashed potatoes.

- Spread the sauerkraut next.

- Finish with shredded cheese on top.

- Put into oven until cheese is golden to brown (about 15–20 minutes).

You can barely mess this dish up–it is so simple. I hope you will enjoy it! The sauerkraut will beautifully help your gut digest what has already been through your digestive system that day. *Guten Appetit!* (German for "Enjoy your meal!")

Week 6, Day 6: More Fermented Foods–Sourdough Starter & Bread

Homemade, warm sourdough bread with a little melted butter and salt is one of my favorite foods on earth. Is your mouth watering too? I have been making my own bread for years, and I have to say, I have gotten quite good at it! However, it took a lot of experimenting to find just the right combination of flour, water, salt, and even bread-container shape that my family finally loves. As with everything new, practice, practice, practice! Even better, get together with a friend and practice making bread together! Beware–once you find the right combination, homemade bread can be addictive! Use common sense and moderation–even when eating your own treats. Let's dive in.

Sourdough Starter Recipe

Takes five days to start from scratch

Directions to make and "feed" the starter:

1. Add 1 cup flour (King Arthur organic bread flour is my favorite) to 1/2 cup filtered water, plus 1 or 2 tablespoons depending on how dry your flour is.

2. Stir, cover with a cloth, and set somewhere out of the way.

3. 24 hours later, divide in half (the half can be used for another starter, or discard).

4. Add 1 cup flour.

5. Add 1/2 cup water plus 1 or 2 tablespoons depending on how dry your flour is.

6. Repeat on day 3.

7. Repeat twice (morning and night) on days 4 and 5.

8. Keep your starter in the fridge until you are ready to use it.

9. If you know someone who already has a sourdough bread starter, ask him or her if you can have two tablespoons, as that is all it takes to make your own batch of sourdough anything!

Sourdough Bread Baking Prep:

- If using a bread bowl, grease with grass-fed butter, ghee (clarified butter), or extra-virgin olive oil.

- If using a baking stone, put flour down under the dough.

- If using a parchment-lined cookie sheet to bake the bread, no greasing or flour is needed.

Sourdough Bread Instructions:

- From 2 cups of your homemade bowl of starter, take out 2 tablespoons for your next batch. Set aside to feed or place in the fridge for up to 2 weeks if you won't use right away.

- Sprinkle about 1/8 cup flour around the edge of the remaining bowl or starter. Lightly work the flour into the starter to create a dough ball.

- Place the dough ball in a greased bread bowl or on baking stone (or parchment paper on a cookie sheet).

- Top with melted butter and mineral salt.

- Bake at 350 degrees Fahrenheit for 40 minutes.

- Let cool for 10 minutes before slicing.

Enjoy yet another fermented food! You can look up recipes online and use your sourdough starter for waffles, muffins, pizza crust, and so much more!

How did your bread turn out the first time you made it? Have patience. It took me a dozen times before I felt like it was perfect. But the taste and health benefits of fresh sourdough bread are worth the effort!

Baking Notes:

_____

_____

_____

_____

_____

Week 6, Day 7: Recap & Reflect

- Your gut houses approximately 80 percent of your immune system.

- Your gut is often referred to as "the second brain."

- Healthy gut bacteria (flora) are killed off from excessive sugar or alcohol consumption, chronic stress, tap water, and antibiotics.

- To replenish healthy gut bacteria, we need to eat approximately three small servings throughout the day (1-2 tablespoons) of fermented foods/beverages per day. Most people don't like the taste of fermented foods at first because we don't eat them enough.

- Fermented foods help your body break down and absorb nutrients, boost your immune system, and keep your bowels regular. Fermented foods also support necessary bacteria in our digestive tract. We need good bacteria on a daily basis to keep the balance of flora in our bodies.

- The best sources of healthy fermented foods and beverages include pickles, pickled vegetables, vinegar, kombucha, kimchi, sourdough and ciabatta bread, and some cultured cheeses.

- Consuming a variety of fermented foods and beverages is essential to getting different types of beneficial bacteria in your gut.

- Try making your own fermented foods and beverages! Remember, if the recipe doesn't work out how you envisioned it the first time, give it another shot!

What did you learn this week?

_____

_____

_____

What surprised you?

_____

_____

_____

What are you excited to implement?

_____

_____

Consuming a variety of fermented foods daily is essential to vibrant health. Detail out an example or two of how you will get three small servings of fermented foods per day:

_____

_____

_____

_____

Did you know there is a connection between your gut and brain health? If you want to learn more about this gut and brain health, check out the book "Gut and Psychology Syndrome" by Dr. Natasha Campbell-McBride MD.

Reflection Notes:

_____

_____

_____

_____

_____

_____

_____

_____

_____

_____

_____

_____

_____

_____

_____

_____

_____

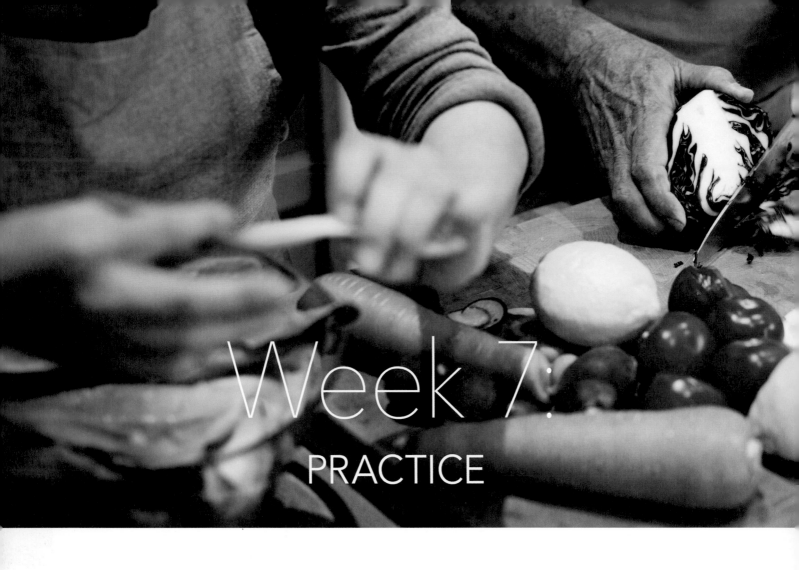

Week 7:
PRACTICE

Welcome to week 7!

Practice makes *progress*. Perfection is *not* our goal. Our goal is to discover God's best for our health and then daily put our knowledge into practice.

**We all make mistakes.
The only failure is not learning
from our mistakes.**

—Dave Gilmore, my dad

Week 7 Action Steps

Number one health goal: _____ *Goal Accomplished!* ☐

Accountability

Record your **strength** workouts in the *Living Wellness Journal;*

weekly goal:_____ _____ (number of days) (minutes per day) ☐

      Partner's goal: _____ _____ (number of days) (minutes per day)

Record your **cardio** workouts in the *Living Wellness Journal;*

weekly goal:_____ _____ (number of days) (minutes per day) ☐

      Partner's goal: _____ _____ ☐

What is your **nutrition** goal this week (remember the SMART goals)? _____

_____ ☐ ☐ ☐ ☐ ☐ ☐ ☐

      Partner's nutrition goal: _____ ☐

Record your **food/beverage** intake in *Living Wellness Journal* or app ☐

Check in with your partner daily. ☐ ☐ ☐ ☐ ☐ ☐

Knowledge

Fill out all questions in this book *prior* to the next meeting. ☐

Mindfulness

Imagine if you were writing your action plan for your child or best friend. Give that same level of care, respect, and love to yourself and your plan for your future. ☐

Inspiration

Pray that the Holy Spirit will inspire you as you complete your Action Plan. ☐

Motivation

Begin with the end in mind as you write your action plan. In a year from now, imagine how you will feel once you complete the action steps in your plan. Remember this future self as you encounter challenges along the way. ☐

Living Wellness Exercises

Do the entire workout multiple times this week! Remember to stretch after your workout.

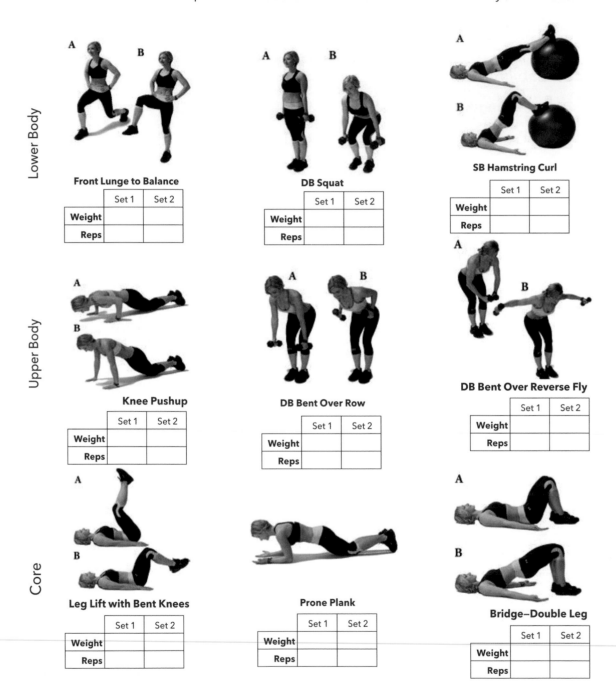

Lower Body

Front Lunge to Balance

	Set 1	Set 2
Weight		
Reps		

DB Squat

	Set 1	Set 2
Weight		
Reps		

SB Hamstring Curl

	Set 1	Set 2
Weight		
Reps		

Upper Body

Knee Pushup

	Set 1	Set 2
Weight		
Reps		

DB Bent Over Row

	Set 1	Set 2
Weight		
Reps		

DB Bent Over Reverse Fly

	Set 1	Set 2
Weight		
Reps		

Core

Leg Lift with Bent Knees

	Set 1	Set 2
Weight		
Reps		

Prone Plank

	Set 1	Set 2
Weight		
Reps		

Bridge–Double Leg

	Set 1	Set 2
Weight		
Reps		

Looking Ahead

This week we will look back at your progress. You will also write your action plan.

Week 7, Day 2: Assessment – Looking Back & Looking Ahead

Look back through week 1 in this book. Read through the Living Wellness Assessment you completed. With a different-colored pen or pencil, make notes of any thoughts or responses that have changed.

Over the course of this journey, how have you grown?

_____

_____

_____

_____

_____

What role does your faith play in your lasting health success?

_____

_____

_____

_____

_____

Please describe everything you ate and drank yesterday with approximate calories (if known):

Food	Calories
Breakfast:	
Snacks:	
Lunch:	
Snacks:	
Dinner:	
Beverages:	
Based on yesterday's account, approximately how many calories are you eating per day?	

Note how your eating habits have changed since week 1.

Do you remember that pesky Excuse Muse? What is the Excuse Muse *still* whispering in your ear? Circle all that still apply:

• I'm too busy • Temptation is too strong • I'm afraid I'll fail • I'm just too tired • I'm not motivated • Bad habits are more fun • I'm distracted • I'm not worth the hassle • I want to get back at someone with my bad choices • My spouse is not worth the work it takes for me to look good • If I lose weight, people who have been nagging me to lose weight will have won

What triggers or harmful habits have you noticed over the past seven weeks?

_____

_____

_____

Make a new plan for overcoming the Excuse Muse, triggers, and harmful habits:

_____

_____

_____

What has been most challenging on this journey?

_____

_____

_____

_____

What have you had an easy time changing?

_____

_____

_____

_____

How Have You Changed?

	A little				Radically
Cardio Exercise					
Strength Exercise					
Vegetables					
Healthy Fats/Oils					
Water					
Fermented Foods/ Beverages					
Reduced Processed Foods					
Reduced Sugar					
Other:					

How Has Your Health Improved?

	A little				Radically
Sleep Quality					
Digestion					
Energy					
Immunity					
Hormones					
Weight					
Brain Clarity					
Other:					
Other:					

PRACTICE

Looking Ahead

Do you believe you are worth the challenge of breaking through tough habits for better health? Why?

_____

_____

_____

What have you learned about yourself on this journey thus far?

_____

_____

_____

What have you learned about God?

_____

_____

_____

God is not finished with us yet!

Do you see God continuing to work in your health and wellness journey? How?

_____

_____

_____

What are your plans to use (or how have you been using) your newfound health to make an impact in your home, community, church, business, school, and the like?

_____

_____

_____

Week 7, Day 3: Action Plan—Mind

You are now going to spend some time writing your action plan. Please give yourself adequate time each day.

Over the last eight weeks, you have been growing deep roots for your health and wellness journey. It's time to grow upward! The action plan includes an assessment of where you are in your mental, physical, and spiritual health. The plan also details your goals, your support team, and what your life will look like once you have implemented your action plan. This plan sets you in motion upward as you begin the next phase of your journey.

Action Plan

Remember, type (or write) your action plan, and make two copies. You will read your action plan out loud at your final small-group meeting. The extra copies will be given to your check-in partner and facilitator. *Refer to the SMART goals when writing this plan.*

Mental and Emotional Health

Before filling out this section, refer back to your mindfulness action steps each week for a reminder about what you have been working on regarding your mental and emotional health. Reflect on what you have been thinking about, struggling with, and excelling at. Use this space to plan and dream for the future.

1. Write out a brief paragraph (personal assessment) of your mental and emotional health (ability to cope with stress, anxiety or depression levels, sleep quality, your self-esteem, keeping your brain active, the health of your closest relationships, etc.).

2. What are your goals to improve your mental and emotional health? List up to three.

    1. Mental/Emotional Health Goal: _____

        Action Step: _____

        Action Step: _____

        Action Step: _____

    2. Mental/Emotional Health Goal: _____

        Action Step: _____

        Action Step: _____

        Action Step: _____

3. Mental/Emotional Health Goal: _____

    Action Step: _____

    Action Step: _____

    Action Step: _____

3. Find a support team. Write down the names of the individuals on your team. Contact them and ask if they will prayerfully consider supporting you on your journey (examples below).

    Counselor or psychologist: _____

    And/Or

    Friend or mentor: _____

4. Write a brief description of exactly what your life will be like when your mental and emotional health improves.

    _____

    _____

    _____

    _____

    _____

    _____

    _____

    _____

    _____

    _____

    _____

Week 7, Day 4: Action Plan—Body

Physical Health

Before filling out this section, refer back to your accountability action steps each week for a reminder about what you have been working on regarding your physical health. Reflect on what you have been thinking about, struggling with, and excelling at. Use this space to plan and dream for the future.

1. Write out a brief paragraph (personal assessment) of your physical health (nutrition, weight, activity level, blood pressure, heart health, sleep quality, energy, immunity, etc.).

_____

_____

_____

_____

_____

_____

2. What are your goals to improve your physical health? List up to three.

   a. Physical Health Goal: _____

      Action Step: _____

      Action Step: _____

      Action Step: _____

   b. Physical Health Goal: _____

      Action Step: _____

      Action Step: _____

      Action Step: _____

   c. Physical Health Goal: _____

      Action Step: _____

      Action Step: _____

      Action Step: _____

3. Find a support team. Write down the names of the individuals on your team. Contact them and ask if they will prayerfully consider supporting you on your journey (examples below).

    Personal trainer or exercise buddy: _____

    And/Or

    Naturopath or nutrition response tester: _____

4. Write a brief description of exactly what your life will be like when your physical health improves.

_____

_____

_____

_____

_____

_____

_____

_____

_____

_____

_____

_____

Week 7, Day 5: Action Plan–Spirit

Spiritual Health

Before filling out this section, refer back to your inspiration action steps each week for a reminder about what you have been working on regarding your spiritual health. Reflect on what you have been thinking about, struggling with, and excelling at. Use this space to plan and dream for the future.

1. Write out a brief paragraph (personal assessment) of your spiritual health (e.g. prayer, reading scripture, church community, attending a Christian conference, listening to a faith-based broadcast, acts of service, fasting, tithing, your relationship with God).

_____

_____

_____

_____

_____

2. What are your goals to improve your spiritual health? List up to three.

    a. Spiritual Health Goal: _____

        Action Step: _____

        Action Step: _____

        Action Step: _____

    b. Spiritual Health Goal: _____

        Action Step: _____

        Action Step: _____

        Action Step: _____

    c. Spiritual Health Goal: _____

        Action Step: _____

        Action Step: _____

        Action Step: _____

3. Find a support team. Write down the names of the individuals on your team. Contact them and ask if they will prayerfully consider supporting you on your journey (examples below).

> Pastor or clergy person: _____
>
> And/Or
>
> Small group or spiritual mentor: _____

4. Write a brief description of exactly what your life will be like when your spiritual health improves.

_____

_____

_____

_____

_____

5. Write out a daily prayer to use as you walk the journey toward better health.

_____

_____

_____

_____

_____

6. In addition to your final check-in partner, share this plan with at least one person from your support team list within one week.

Person with whom you will share your plan: _____

Personal Action Plan adapted from *Journey to Freedom* by Scott Reall

Week 7, Day 6: Overcoming Challenges and Setbacks

Think about the stages of change that we studied in the first week. Do you remember the stages?

Pre-contemplation

Contemplation

Preparation

Action

Maintenance

Relapse

Another word for *relapse* is *setback*. How do you plan to get back on track after encountering setbacks?

_____

_____

_____

_____

_____

_____

_____

_____

_____

_____

_____

_____

_____

_____

_____

_____

_____

Week 7, Day 7: Recap & Reflect

Use this space to write out/compile your completed action plan or type it up. Please bring a copy for your final check-in partner and another for your facilitator(s) for future encouragement.

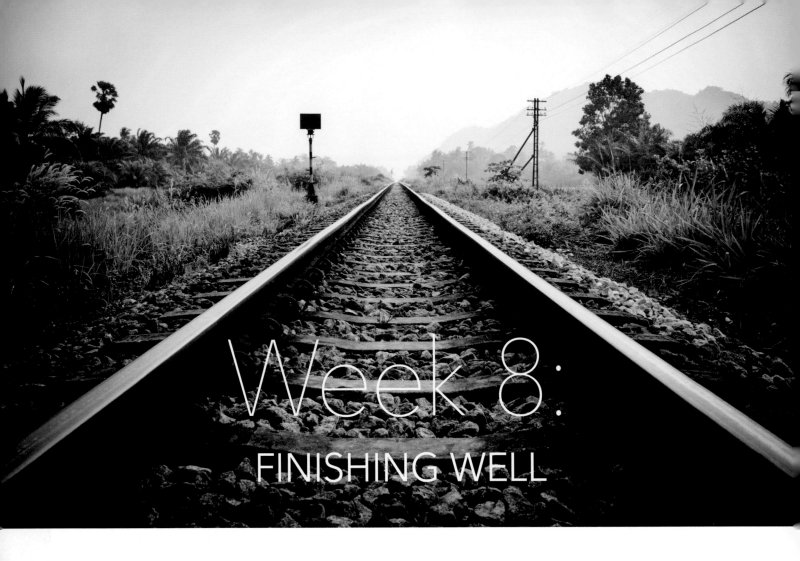

Week 8:
FINISHING WELL

Finishing Well & Breaking through the Health Barrier—Our final week together!

Welcome to our final week! Job well done on completing the book. You have likely grown more than you realize. Celebrate your accomplishments and all that you have been working on in the past eight weeks! We are excited for you to enter into the next phase of your health journey.

Philippians 1:6 reminds us that
"And I am certain that God, who began the good work within you, will continue his work until it is finally finished on the day when Christ Jesus returns. (NLT)"

- Philippians 1:6 (NLT)

Week 8 Action Steps

Number one health goal: _____ *Goal Accomplished!* ☐

1. Exchange your action plan with your check-in partner from last week.
2. Check in with your partner daily. ☐ ☐ ☐ ☐ ☐ ☐ ☐
3. Read through your action plan on a regular basis and implement it.
4. Remember to celebrate your successes.

Congratulations on getting to this point in your journey! You have traveled long to get here, and yet your journey continues. We never really "arrive" at health, until the day we meet our Creator. Rather, we just continue learning and making decisions that bring us closer to the person we were created to be.

Change takes time. You may only be two months into your transformation. Think back to when you (or someone you know) learned how to ride a bicycle. How can you forget, right? If you were like me, it was hard work, painful, and often frustrating, especially if you had an older sibling who was beyond your skills and enjoyed pointing out your shortcomings in learning.

Once you practiced and became comfortable on the bike, you could take one hand off the bike, one foot off the bike, close your eyes for a moment or two, and then eventually you just felt free—free to ride without a care in the world, free to know you were confident on the bike when you steered, when you turned, and when you rode over an unexpected bump. I remember the feeling of freedom so clearly since that moment. The pain and work of learning how to ride my bike paid off. Have I fallen off and gotten hurt since? Yes. If I could go back, I would do it all over again for the exhilarating freedom of riding my bike. The falls become less frequent with time and practice, and enjoyment of the activity grows. I loved (and still love) riding my bike, it's my happy movement, but it took a lot of hard work and discipline to enjoy the freedom I have now.

Our health journeys are similar to learning how to ride a bike. In the beginning, there is uncertainty, doubt, pain, struggle, and perceived failure. But as with most journeys, eventually there is knowledge, mindfulness, inspiration, accountability, and motivation. Having an awareness of these elements empowers you to make consistent, wise decisions. There is freedom in discipline. I am not talking about a strict set of rules or a "do this" and "do not do that" approach to health and wellness. I am talking about a lifestyle. I was purposeful to use language like "try this" and "avoid that." Food is not evil. Exercise doesn't have to be painful. *Discipline* is not a dirty word.

The more we learn and practice disciplining our bodies, minds, and spirits, the stronger they become and the more freedom we gain. I want to be free. Do you want to be free?

_____

_____

_____

Do you want to count calories every day for the rest of your life?

No, probably not.

Do you want to look at every food label for the rest of your life?

No, that is too time-consuming.

Do you want to avoid restaurants forever because you cannot handle temptations and the thought of making terrible choices scare you? No, I hope not.

My prayer and desire is that *Living Wellness for Growth Groups* has guided you in this phase of your health journey and that it's enabled you to confidently make statements like *I know my body's needs, the signs of hunger and thirst, and the nutrients I need to be balanced from the inside out. I confidently walk through the grocery store with freedom, plan my meals with ease, and eat out with friends and family when I want. I practice happy movement because I feel better when I exercise, and I know it's vital to my health.* This is freedom. It comes with practice and discipline. Agreeing with God that your health is important and freely becoming a good steward of your body allows health to become a joyful journey.

 Alongside freedom comes the reward of health. Were any of your goals to feel better, look better, have more energy, have less pain, sleep better, have less disease, be more confident, and achieve and maintain a healthy weight?

Did you begin to make significant progress toward those goals? Have you made a breakthrough yet? Are you healthier now than when you started? Did you set out on your trip with appropriate goals, adequate support, and a backup plan for setbacks? If you did, you are now eating better, moving more, feeling better, and you have likely improved your physical health and your weight. If you are not there yet, don't panic. Don't even feel disappointed! Shame has no place here. Keep moving forward.

Think about the child learning to ride a bicycle as if it were your child. What if he or she practiced for days and weeks and still couldn't figure out how to ride? What would you tell the child? *I guess riding a bike just isn't for you. Try again when you're less busy. I guess you were just born that way; time to accept it.* No! You would encourage; offer suggestions; say, "Practice again;" believe in; help and guide; and then celebrate in his or her success. *You are somewhere on that bicycle-learning curve!* Now is not the time to stop riding. It's not the time to put the road map down. Keep practicing your part in health to receive a breakthrough, no matter where you are in your journey.

The following excerpt is from Mark Batterson's book *The Circle Maker* on the challenge of breakthrough:

> I had the privilege of hearing Chuck Yeager recount his experiences at the Smithsonian National Air and Space Museum with Parker's Cub Scout troop. Right outside the IMAX theater where Yeager gave the speech, the Bell X-1 is symbolically suspended in midair, along with other historic aircraft and spacecraft. Each one represents a breakthrough. Each one is a testament to the ingenuity and irrepressibility of the human spirit, which of course, is a gift of the Holy Spirit.
>
> Just like the sound barrier, there is a faith barrier. And breaking the faith barrier in the spiritual realm is much like breaking the sound barrier in the physical realm. If you want to experience a supernatural breakthrough, it often feels like you're about to lose control, about to fall apart. That is when you need to press in and pray through. If you allow them to, your disappointments will create drag. If you allow them to, your doubts will nosedive your dreams. But if you pray through, God will come through and you'll experience supernatural breakthrough.

This parallel of breaking through a sound barrier and a spiritual barrier is a powerful illustration. Think about those astronauts preparing to launch into space. There was fear, excitement, anticipation, and thoughts of the unknown. Once the 1,607,185 pounds of solid rocket boosters were ignited, there was an unbelievable amount of noise, pressure, and trembling. Imagine yourself in the launch seat! Have you allowed the challenge and the pressure of your health efforts to prevail? Have you offered your fear up to God and do you have faith that there will be a breakthrough? If so, wow, what a journey!

Breakthroughs are scary, but they precede freedom and better health. Breakthroughs bring an ease and comfort, knowing you worked hard, believed in yourself, and achieved something worthwhile. With God's help, anything is possible. If you are feeling the pressure of the engines and the awareness of uncertainty, press in, pray, and have faith. A breakthrough is up ahead.

Remember, there will be setbacks as we continue along, but they *do not define you*, and they do not have to derail you. Setbacks are a part of the journey. Embrace them, learn from them, and then ask the Creator of the universe, our father in heaven, to strengthen you and continue moving your life in the direction toward fullness and abundance.

Do you believe you are worth the challenge of breaking through tough habits, perhaps even lifelong habits, for better health? Please explain.

_____

_____

_____

Review this book often. The more you bring health to the front of your mind, the more your wellness becomes a top priority. You now know what to do to be a healthier person. Practicing consistent healthy habits makes for a lifetime of improvement. Think how often parents must remind children to brush their teeth when they are young! After 999,999 times, I think my children finally understand the importance, and they do it without thinking (although occasionally they still need reminding). We, too, need reminding. We need to hold one another accountable and hold one another up to a standard above average, because right now, there is nothing healthy about average health.

Do you believe you are worth exceptional health of your mind, body, and spirit?

You are worth it! I know you are worth it. You were created to live an abundant life. You are created for more than mediocre.

You are the most beautiful creation God has ever made. Let us accept the gift of our bodies and be excited for the amazing journey ahead.

May God richly bless you on your continued journey,

Ashley R. Darkenwald

Reflection Notes:

_____

_____

_____

_____

_____

_____

_____

_____

_____

_____

_____

_____

_____

_____

_____

_____

_____

_____

_____

_____

_____

_____

_____

_____

APPENDIX & RESOURCES

Appendix A

Kombucha Brewing Instructions Using a Full-Size SCOBY

Supplies:

Teakettle or pot
1-gallon glass container
3 quarts of purified water (no chlorine)
1 cup of sugar—organic cane sugar works well (no stevia or xylitol)
4–5 tea bags or 4–5 teaspoons loose-leaf tea
1–2 cups of starter liquid (kombucha tea)
SCOBY (symbiotic colony of bacteria and yeast)
Tightly woven cloth cover & rubber band (no cheesecloth)

Brewing Recipe:

Makes 1 gallon of kombucha

1. Heat 4 cups of purified water in a teakettle or pot.

2. Just as the water starts to boil, turn off heat and let cool 1–2 minutes, then add to your brewing vessel. Make sure the vessel isn't too cold or it could crack.

3. Add 4–5 tea bags (green, black, or a combo). Steep 5–10 minutes.

4. Remove the tea bags and stir in 1 cup of sugar until dissolved.

5. Add 2 quarts (8 cups) of purified water; this should bring the temperature of the boiled water down to lukewarm (test with food thermometer). Ideal temp = 75–85 degrees Fahrenheit. You may need to let your liquid sit for a while to cool further.

6. Add SCOBY and starter liquid. (In future batches, retain 1 to 2 cups from your brew to use as starter liquid.)

7. Cover container with a tightly woven cloth and rubber band.

8. Place the container in a dark, warm, ventilated area for 7 to 21 days (depending on taste, temperature, etc.). Keep out of direct sunlight. It may or may not get fizzy. The SCOBY may rise to the top or sink to the bottom—it doesn't matter; the new culture will always form at the top.

9. When you are ready to test your kombucha, take a straw and gently slide it beneath the new SCOBY and have a sip. When it has the right balance of sour and sweet, then it is ready. Allow at least 3 brewing cycles for the SCOBY to integrate into its new environment before dividing it.

Bottling:

1. With sanitized hands or a ladle, remove the culture(s) and place in a clean bowl.

2. Ladle or pour 1 to 2 cups of liquid from the top of the brew over the cultures. This will serve as starter liquid for the next batch.

3. Cover cultures with a cloth and set aside.

4. Find clean bottles with tight-fitting lids. Recycled bottles are fine, but avoid metal lids that may corrode. Flip tops are recommended.

5. If flavoring the kombucha, place fruit/juice/flowers/spices directly into the bottles. A little goes a long way. Experiment with different flavors that sound good to you.

6. Place the bottles in the sink, insert a funnel in the first bottle, and ladle or pour in the kombucha.

7. Repeat for the rest of the bottles, straining the yeast if you prefer. Tighten the lids and set aside 1 to 3 days, burping the bottles each day to release excess carbonation and prevent explosions.

8. Move bottles to the fridge as they reach the desired carbonation/flavor. This halts fermentation occurring due to flavorings.

Recipe and bottling modified from Kombucha Camp

Bone Broth Recipe

Recipe from Kelley Suggs, CHES, founder of Lithe Wellness Solutions

Ingredients:

Bones of 1 chicken *or* turkey, *or* soup pack of beef bones, *or* venison or other wild game
Leftover trimmings from carrots, onions, celery, and garlic
2 tablespoons of acidic medium, such as vinegar, whey, or lemon juice
Enough water to cover
1 tablespoon of salt
½ teaspoon of pepper
Spices and herbs to flavor it to satisfy your taste buds. Good combinations include 2-3 sprigs fresh or 2 teaspoons dried parsley, thyme, and dill and two cloves of garlic.

Directions:

1. Place all ingredients in the slow cooker, cover with water, and cook on low for 24-48 hours. Add additional water if necessary.

2. Cook until you can sink the nail of your thumb into a bone. Strain out all the solid pieces and throw them away.

3. Use within a week or freeze in 2-cup increments.

Benefits: powerhouse of nutrition; easy to digest; full of gelatin, vitamins, and minerals; no chemicals; no MSG (very difficult for a person to work through when his or her immune system is already working really, really hard).

Appendix B

Ashley's Weekly Food-Prep Routine Example

Below is an example of my morning prep routine. I usually tackle this list *once* per week—or I break the list up throughout the week as my schedule allows.

Prep Time: About 90 minutes

Serves: You and your loved ones!

- [ ] Make or bottle kombucha
- [ ] Soak seeds, nuts, beans, and grains
- [ ] Make homemade trail mix
- [ ] Make bone broth
- [ ] Bake or boil hard-boiled eggs
- [ ] Wash fruits and vegetables and dry well; slice and store in fridge
- [ ] Wash vegetables like carrots, celery, and peppers; slice and store in fridge
- [ ] Peel ripe bananas; store and freeze
- [ ] Make or feed sourdough starter (sourdough must be cared for daily or placed in fridge to keep fresh)
- [ ] Put something in the slow cooker

Appendix C

Five Protein-Packed Recipes

Chicken Braised in Liquid Aminos* and Lemon Juice

Serves 4

> Coconut aminos*
> Cayenne pepper flakes
> 1 clove garlic
> Extra-virgin olive oil
> Organic cane sugar
> 1 lemon
> 1-pound bone-in chicken (nitrite- and nitrate-free)

Brown bone-in chicken pieces in a few tablespoons of extra-virgin olive oil. Remove and stir in 1 tablespoon chopped garlic. Add the minced zest of a lemon, a pinch of cayenne, 2 tablespoons aminos, 1 teaspoon organic cane sugar,** and 1/3 cup water; stir. Add the chicken, cover, and simmer. Turn the pieces once; the dish will be done in about 15 minutes. Add lemon juice and coconut aminos to taste.

*Coconut aminos are a soy sauce alternative.

**Organic cane sugar is an excellent alternative to table sugar. It is dehydrated cane juice, sweet and packed with nutrients.

Grilled Chicken with Pesto Sauce

Serves 4

  2 cups fresh basil
  1 clove garlic
  Sea salt and pepper
  Pine nuts
  Parmesan cheese
  Extra-virgin olive oil
  1-pound chicken cutlets (nitrite- and nitrate-free)

To make the pesto, puree 2 cups fresh basil, 1 garlic clove, a pinch of sea salt, 2 tablespoons pine nuts, 1/2 cup grated Parmesan, and 1/2 cup extra-virgin olive oil in a blender or food processor.

Season 1-pound chicken cutlets with sea salt and pepper. Grill them, turning once, about 8 minutes total. Paint chicken with pesto and serve.

Stir-Fried Spicy Beef

Serves 4

  1-pound flank steak
  1/2 cup basil
  1 clove garlic
  Unrefined coconut oil
  Red pepper flakes
  Coconut aminos
  1 lime or lemon

Thinly slice 1 pound of flank steak across the grain into bite-size pieces. Chop 1/2 cup basil and mix with beef; set aside. Cook 1 1/2 tablespoons minced garlic in 1 tablespoon of coconut oil until slightly brown.

Add beef-basil mixture and 1/4 tablespoon red pepper flakes; cook for 2 minutes. Add 1 tablespoon aminos and the juice of half a lime or lemon and serve.

Chicken with Citrus Glaze

Serves 4

- 2 lemons
- 1 orange
- 1 grapefruit
- Extra-virgin olive oil
- 1 clove garlic
- Fresh thyme leaves
- Sea salt and pepper
- 1 small onion
- 4 boneless chicken breasts (nitrite- and nitrate-free)

To make the sauce, warm the zest and juice of one lemon, plus the sections of another lemon, an orange, and a grapefruit in a pan. Add 1/4 cup olive oil, 1 teaspoon fresh thyme leaves, 1/2 teaspoon minced garlic, one small minced onion, sea salt, and pepper. Rub boneless chicken with olive oil and sprinkle with sea salt and pepper. Broil or grill. Serve with the citrus sauce.

Chicken Tikka with Greek Yogurt Sauce

Serves 4

- Low sugar, plain Greek yogurt
- Ground almonds or walnuts
- 4 boneless chicken breasts (nitrite- and nitrate-free)
- 1 clove garlic
- Spices: cardamom, coriander, ginger, sea salt, and pepper

Cut boneless chicken into 1-inch chunks. Combine with 1/4 cup low-sugar, plain Greek yogurt, 1/4 cup ground almonds or walnuts, and 1 teaspoon each ground cardamom, ground coriander, minced ginger, and minced garlic. Remove chicken from the marinade and grill until brown and cooked through. To make the sauce, mix 1 cup yogurt with 1 teaspoon minced garlic and some lemon juice, salt, and pepper. Serve with the chicken.

Appendix D

Grocery List for Meal Planning

The first time I went into a boutique, organic grocery store, I walked out with a $300+ bill, and I cried all the way home. The worst part was when I put everything away and my kids came home, and they opened the pantry and said, "There's nothing to eat!" I think I cried some more. I can't remember all the details because I blocked it out.

I hope you have not had a similar experience, but if you have, please don't let one or two expensive experiences deter you from shopping to *nourish* your body.

Navigating the grocery store can be an enjoyable experience. Make a list (or use the sample list below), shop the perimeter of the store (when applicable), read labels, and overhaul your pantry and fridge one section at a time, not all at once (unless you have the means to do so)! Over time, you will be a completely different shopper.

Beverages—herbal tea, water, sparkling water, kombucha, and so on

-
-
-
-

Bread/bakery—100 percent whole-grain items (sprouted when available)

-
-
-
-

Canned/jarred goods—vegetables, spaghetti sauce, fruit, almond butter, ketchup (avoid additives)

-
-
-
-

Dairy—butter, cheeses, eggs, milk, yogurt (from raw, organic, pasture-raised animals when available)

-

-

-

-

-

Dry/baking goods—rice, beans, nuts

-

-

-

-

-

Frozen foods—meat, vegetables, fruit

-

-

-

-

-

Meat—fish, poultry, beef, pork (avoid preservatives)

-

-

-

-

-

Produce—fruits, vegetables (organic when available)

-
-
-
-
-

Household products (what you use in use in home and on your body is important—choose the most natural household products available)

-
-
-
-
-

Cleaners—all-purpose laundry detergent, dish washing liquid/detergent (look for brands like Norwex with no fillers)

-
-
-
-
-

Paper goods—paper towels, toilet paper, aluminum foil, sandwich bags

-
-
-
-

Personal care—shampoo, soap, hand soap, shaving cream (avoid carcinogens like ethanolamines and parabens)

-
-
-
-
-

Other—baby items, pet items, batteries, greeting cards, and the like

-
-
-
-
-
-
-
-
-
-
-
-
-
-
-
-
-

FOSS Chart Health Continuum

Transform your pantry. Transform your health.

*FOSS chart adapted from the Westin A. Price Foundation Shopping Guide Categories

FOSS	Processed Food (Toxic)–Avoid	Less Processed (Some Health Benefits)	Unprocessed (Nourishing)– Enjoy in Moderation	Enjoy with Reckless Abandon
Flour & Grains	Enriched flour Bleached flour Bulgur White flour products Puffed grain products, such as rice cakes Factory-made modern soy foods Soybeans, unless used for making fermented foods like natto Soybean sprouting seeds and sprouts Alfalfa seeds and sprouts	100 percent whole grains Unsoaked granola Dried beans and lentils Unsoaked whole-grain rice Canned beans Buckwheat, corn, and brown rice pasta Organic white rice	Soaked and/or sprouted grains; fermented grains, such as sourdough Organic dried beans and lentils Soaked and/or sprouted 100 percent whole grains and whole-grain breakfast cereals that must be cooked Wild rice Organic popcorn (to pop at home) Organic sprouting seeds except alfalfa and soybean	Nothing except the love of Jesus!
Oils & Fats	Partially hydrogenated oils Most commercial vegetable oils, including cottonseed, soy, corn, canola, rice bran, hemp, and grapeseed oils All margarines, spreads, and partially hydrogenated vegetable shortenings	Pasteurized grass-fed butter Cold-pressed or expeller-pressed sesame, sunflower, peanut, macadamia, avocado, almond, walnut, pecan, pistachio, hazelnut, pumpkin seed, and high-oleic safflower oils in small amounts Refined palm oil Refined coconut oil Extra-virgin olive oil Cold-pressed flaxseed oil	Raw grass-fed butter, organic cold-pressed flaxseed oil, extra-virgin sesame oil, red palm oil Organic extra-virgin olive oil Organic cold-pressed macadamia, avocado, almond, high-oleic sunflower, and high-oleic safflower oils Organic unrefined virgin coconut oil Unrefined organic palm oil Fat and lard from pigs allowed to graze Tallow and suet from grass-fed cows and sheep Poultry fat from pastured poultry	It's a fallacy that you can eat endless amounts of anything.

FOSS	Processed Food (Toxic)–Avoid	Less Processed (Some Health Benefits)	Unprocessed (Nourishing)– Enjoy in Moderation	Enjoy with Reckless Abandon
Sugar	White sugar, corn syrup, high fructose corn syrup, yacon syrup, imitation syrups, stevia extracts (powder) Artificial sweeteners, such as sucralose (Splenda) and aspartame (NutraSweet and Equal); sugar alcohols, such as xylitol	Organic sugar in the raw Organic jams Heated honey Brown rice syrup Organic blue agave Jams made with organic sugar Concentrated fruit juices Organic liquid stevia	Organic fruit Organic natural sweeteners, such as molasses, green stevia leaves and green stevia powder, dehydrated sugar cane juice, malt syrups, coconut sugar, palm sugar, date sugar, and sorghum syrup Maple syrup, maple sugar Raw honey, preferably unfiltered	The key to long-term health success is:
Salt	Table salt, sodium nitrite, sodium nitrate Monosodium glutamate (MSG)	Kosher salt Commercial sea salt	Unrefined mineral salt, such as Celtic sea salt or pink Himalayan (generally, salt should have a color)	MODERATION

EWG Shopper's Guide to Pesticides in Produce

Dirty Dozen (*always* buy organic)	Clean Fifteen (OK to eat nonorganic)
Apples	Avocados
Peaches	Sweet corn
Nectarines	Pineapple
Strawberries	Cabbage
Grapes	Sweet peas–frozen
Celery	Onions
Spinach	Asparagus
Sweet bell peppers	Mangoes
Cucumbers	Papayas
Cherry tomatoes	Kiwi
Snap peas–imported	Eggplant
Potatoes	Grapefruit
	Cantaloupe
	Cauliflower
	Sweet potatoes

Appendix E

Bristol Stool Chart

	Bristol Stool Chart	
Type 1		Separate hard lumps; very constipated
Type 2		Lumpy and sausage-like; slightly constipated
Type 3		Sausage-shaped with cracks on the surface; healthy
Type 4		Sausage- or snake-like, smooth and soft; healthy
Type 5		Soft blobs with clear-cut edges; lacking fiber
Type 6		Fluffy pieces with mushy edges; inflammation
Type 7		Watery, entirely liquid; inflammation

Appendix F

Serving Size Suggestion for Fruits

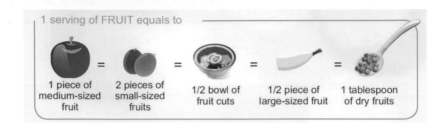

Protein Sources ~ Serving Size ~ Grams of Protein

Food	Serving Size	Approximate Grams of Protein
Free-range chicken	3 ounces (deck of cards)	27
Grass-fed hamburger	3 ounces	22
Wild-caught fish	3 ounces	22
Lentils, cooked	½ cup (tennis ball)	17
Kidney beans, cooked	½ cup	8
Raw milk	1 cup (fist)	8
Plain yogurt	1 cup	8
Hard cheese	1 ounce (tip of thumb)	7
Free-range egg	1 large	6
Raw mixed nuts	1 ounce	5

Appendix G

Mindful Eating Instructions

1. Look within. *Am I hungry? Am I thirsty? Will food satisfy my hunger? What will nourish me in this moment?* Accept your choice.

2. Ask your body what it wants and *listen. Often,* we are afraid that our bodies will choose cookies and doughnuts, but your body is a complex instrument, and many times if you listen, you will know what you need.

3. Eat with awareness: taste, savor, sense how it makes your body feel. Slow down to chew and taste your food. Have you ever really eaten? Inattention leaves us hungry. We hunger for the experience. Transform your relationship with food.

4. Listen for feedback. Sit back and relax. Breathe. Did the meal satisfy you? Would you eat differently next time? Experience the effects of your body after a full meal. Use experience as a teacher.

5. Release your thoughts about food. Move on. Be free from thinking of food for a while. Inability to release thoughts about food is at the root of our most challenging eating habits. Moving away from thoughts about food gives us the freedom to direct mental and emotional energy toward God's best for our lives.

*Mindful eating tips from The Institute for Psychology of Eating

Appendix H

Additional Resources by Topic

Below are some of my favorite books. This is not an exhaustive list; there are so many other fantastic resources available. These are just a few authors that have mentored me on my journey. I hope you enjoy them as much as I have.

Change

Prochaska, James O., John C. Norcross, and Carlo C. DiClemente. *Changing for Good: The Revolutionary Program That Explains the Six Stages of Change and Teaches You How to Free Yourself from Bad Habits.*

Thompson, Curt. *Anatomy of the Soul: Surprising Connections between Neuroscience and Spiritual Practices That Can Transform Your Life and Relationships.*

Children's Health

Campbell-McBride, Dr. Natasha. *Gut and Psychology Syndrome.*

Compart, Pamela and Dana Laake. *The Kid-Friendly ADHD & Autism Cookbook, Updated and Revised: The Ultimate Guide to the Gluten-Free, Casein-Free Diet.*

Cookbooks

Compart, Pamela and Dana Laake. *The Kid-Friendly ADHD & Autism Cookbook, Updated and Revised: The Ultimate Guide to the Gluten-Free, Casein-Free Diet.*

Fallon, Sally and Mary Enig. *Nourishing Traditions: The Cookbook that Challenges Politically Correct Nutrition and the Diet Dictocrats.*

Leake, Lisa. *100 Days of Real Food.*

Walker, Danielle. *Against All Grain.*

Disease Prevention

Somers, Suzanne. *TOX-SICK: From Toxic to Not Sick.*

Fats and Oils

Bowden, Jonny and Stephen Sinatra. *The Great Cholesterol Myth*.

Enig, Dr. Mary G. *Know Your Fats: The Complete Primer for Understanding the Nutrition of Fats, Oils and Cholesterol.*.

Erasmus, Udo. *Fats That Heal, Fats That Kill: The Complete Guide to Fats, Oils, Cholesterol and Human Health*.

Finances

Ramsey, Dave. *Dave Ramsey's Complete Guide to Money*

Grains

Perlmutter, David. *Grain Brain: The Surprising Truth about Wheat, Carbs, and Sugar—Your Brain's Silent Killers*.

Walker, Danielle. *Against All Grain*.

Leadership

Detrick, Jodi. *The Jesus-Hearted Woman: 10 Leadership Qualities for Enduring and Endearing Influence*.

Milk

Woodford, Keith (foreword by Thomas Cowan). *Devil in the Milk: Illness, Health and the Politics of A1 and A2 Milk*.

Nutrition

Bowden, Jonny. *150 Healthiest Foods on Earth*.

Bowden, Jonny and Stephen Sinatra. *The Great Cholesterol Myth*.

Darkenwald, Ashley. *Living Wellness: The inFIT Approach to Proven Weight Loss and Dynamic Nutrition*.

Fallon, Sally and Mary Enig. *Nourishing Traditions: The Cookbook that Challenges Politically Correct Nutrition and the Diet Dictocrats*.

Price, Weston A. *Nutrition and Physical Degeneration*.

Spiritual Growth

Chambers, Oswald. *My Utmost for His Highest.*

Corbett, Steve and Brian Fikkert. *Helping without Hurting in Short-Term Missions.*

Diederich, F. Remy. *Healing the Hurts of Your Past: A Guide to Overcoming the Pain of Shame.*

Meyer, Joyce. *Beauty for Ashes.*

Peterson, Eugene. *A Long Obedience in the Same Direction: Discipleship in an Instant Society.*

Piper, John. *Hunger for God.*

Reall, Scott. *Journey to Freedom.*

Terkeurst, Lysa. *Made to Crave.*

Thompson, Curt. *Anatomy of the Soul: Surprising Connections between Neuroscience and Spiritual Practices That Can Transform Your Life and Relationships.*

Appendix I

Ashley's Favorite Kitchen Tools

Having a few trusted tools saves you time and money in the kitchen. Below are a few of my favorites (in order of my most frequently used tools):

Sharp knives
Small blender or bullet-style chopper
Kitchen scissors
Mandolin slicer
Lots of canning jars of all sizes (get rid of old plastic containers!)
Soaking/sprouting jar with mesh lid
Slow cooker
Steamer or rice cooker
Garlic press
Apple slicer
Wok
Waffle maker
Dehydrator
Toaster oven
Spiralizer
Juicer
Food processor (I can do most everything I need in my small blender, but if you have it in the budget, a food processor or heavy-duty blender is a wonderful, time-saving kitchen tool.)
Old-fashioned juice press

Appendix J

Borg Rating of Perceived Exertion (RPE) Scale

While doing physical activity, we want you to rate your perception of your exertion. This feeling should reflect how heavy and strenuous the exercise feels to you, combining all sensations and feelings of physical stress, effort, and fatigue. Do not concern yourself with any one factor such as leg pain or shortness of breath, but try to focus on your total feeling of exertion.

Look at the rating scale below while you are engaging in an activity; the scale ranges from 6 to 20, where 6 means "no exertion at all" and 20 means "maximal exertion." Choose the number from below that best describes your level of exertion. This will give you a good idea of the intensity level of your activity, and you can use this information to speed up or slow down your movements to reach your desired range. If you are not wearing a heart rate monitor, this scale is useful to determine if you are practicing cardiovascular exercise or physical activity (see week 1). Cardiovascular exercise occurs approximately at an exertion of 13 or more.

Try to appraise your feeling of exertion as honestly as possible without thinking about what the actual physical load is. Your own feeling of effort and exertion is important, not how it compares to others. Look at the scale and the expression and then give a number.

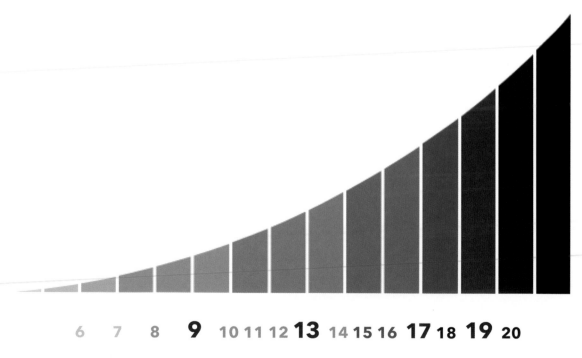

6 7 8 **9** 10 11 12 **13** 14 15 16 **17** 18 **19** 20

NO EXERTION AT ALL   MAXIMAL EXERTION

9 corresponds to "very light" exercise. For a healthy person, it is comparable to walking slowly at his or her own pace for some minutes.

13 on the scale is "somewhat hard" exercise, but it still feels ok to continue.

17 is "very hard," meaning very strenuous. A healthy person can still go on, but he or she really has to push him- or herself. It feels very heavy, and the person is very tired. Examples of this exertion are kettlebells, trail racing, or intense rowing.

19 on the scale is an extremely strenuous exercise level. For most people this is the most strenuous exercise they have ever experienced. Labor and delivery, or sprinting for extended periods of time are examples of this level of exertion.

Borg RPE scale © Gunnar Borg, 1970, 1985, 1994, 1998

Appendix K

Thirteen Steps to Climb a Mountain (Just for fun)

The front cover picture is Pikes Peak in Colorado. I hiked these mountains with dear friend and mentor Tracy Shearer many years ago, when God gave me the inspiration for the title *Living Wellness*. At the airport and on the plane ride back to Minnesota, Tracy and I wrote on beverage napkins and paper tablecloths about health being more than just a set of rules or the latest diet. *Living Wellness* is a journey. I hope you have had a mountaintop experience at some point in the last eight weeks. If not, here are some instructions on how to climb a mountain. Bring a friend and discover your journey to living wellness.

1. Do your research.

2. Assess your physical and mental strength.

3. Get fit.

4. Acquire your tools.

5. Learn about mountaineering ethics.

6. Get training.

7. Plan your first climb.

8. Keep improving your skills and trying harder mountain climbs.

9. Find a trustworthy, experienced guide.

10. Prepare for the trip.

11. Understand what's involved on arrival at the mountain.

12. On belay (begin climbing).

13. Descend with a plan.

Original "How to Climb a Mountain" accessed from WikiHow online.

Appendix L

To perform the exercises in this book, I recommend the following equipment:

- A stability (exercise) ball (55–75 centimeters)
- 3 pairs of dumbbells: light, medium, and heavy
- A foam roller (you can use a tennis ball or rolling pin if you are on a budget)

Do you belong to a gym? If so, it should have these tools. If you plan to buy equipment and work out on your own, use this guideline for dumbbells. Start with a moderate weight dumbbell, 8–12 pounds for women and 12–20 pounds for men. Perform dumbbell biceps curls and count how many you can do.

If you can do more than 16–20 repetitions (reps) *without arching or leaning back*, this will be your light pair of dumbbells. If you can do between 12–16 reps, this is your medium pair; buy one pair the next heavier weight and one pair the next lighter weight from your original medium pair of dumbbells. If you can do at most between 6–12 repetitions, this is your heavy pair; buy two additional pairs (two weight selections lighter than your heavy pair). These exercise tools are excellent to start you on your fitness journey.

Living Wellness Strength Training Routine

This proven workout includes exercises that promote stabilization and strength. You can work out every day, but be sure to give your muscles forty-eight hours of rest between strength workouts for adequate repair before working the same muscle group again. For example, if you perform upper-body exercises on Monday, wait until Wednesday to do upper-body exercises again.

Perform the full workout circuit style with one exercise from each row (lower body, upper body, and core) with minimal rest between exercises. Repeat the pattern with the next column. You can go through the warm-up, all nine exercises, and stretching one time (one set) in approximately twenty to twenty-five minutes. If you want to increase your strength gains faster, or you want to focus on a specific muscle group, keep repeating the exercises of your choice to complete additional sets. The more you work your muscles, the faster you will see definition and weight loss results. If you have not worked out in at least a month, set small, attainable goals such as working out one to two times per week. Developing lasting habits is much easier when your goals are realistic and your practice is consistent. You can always increase your exercise with time, but it is more difficult to get back on the path if you become burned out or injured.

Living Wellness Workout Guidelines

The goal is to fatigue (exhaust the muscle) after no more than twenty repetitions (reps). If you can do more than twenty reps per exercise, increase your weight or resistance.

We will break down this whole workout in pieces over the next eight weeks, but if you want to get a head start, use the instructions below.

First time (set) through: Warm up. Go through all the exercises slowly, 15–20 repetitions (reps) each, with no resistance (no weight), 3–5 minutes.

Second set: Perform the exercises one at a time, with resistance when appropriate, starting with one lower-body exercise, one upper-body exercise, and one core exercise with minimal rest in between. Perform all nine exercises and then repeat as your fitness goals and time permit!

This workout is designed to build your body's stabilization endurance and core strength and to prepare you for more challenging moves in the future. Take your time working through the exercises. Usually, slower is better (and safer too).

Remember to stretch your muscles, as stretching is as important as the workout itself.

Living Wellness Workout 1

First time (set) through: Warm up. Go through all of the exercises slowly, 15-20 repetitions (reps) each, with no resistance (no weight), 3-5 minutes. **Second set:** Perform the exercises one at a time, with resistance when appropriate, starting with one lower body exercise, one upper body exercise, and one core exercise with minimal rest in between. Perform all nine exercises and then repeat as your fitness goals and time permit! Phase I is designed to build your body's stabilization endurance, core strength, and to prepare you for more challenging moves in the future. Take your time working through the exercises. Usually, slower is better (and safer, too). Remember to stretch your muscles as stretching is as important as the workout itself.

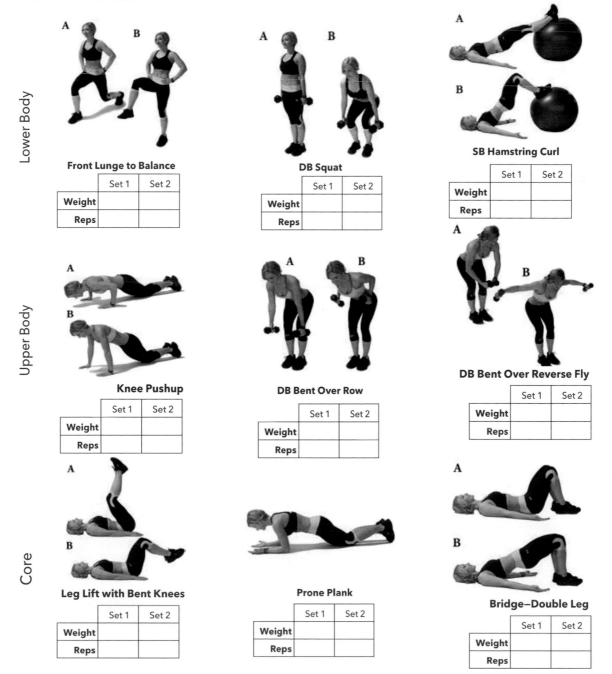

Lower Body

Front Lunge to Balance

	Set 1	Set 2
Weight		
Reps		

DB Squat

	Set 1	Set 2
Weight		
Reps		

SB Hamstring Curl

	Set 1	Set 2
Weight		
Reps		

Upper Body

Knee Pushup

	Set 1	Set 2
Weight		
Reps		

DB Bent Over Row

	Set 1	Set 2
Weight		
Reps		

DB Bent Over Reverse Fly

	Set 1	Set 2
Weight		
Reps		

Core

Leg Lift with Bent Knees

	Set 1	Set 2
Weight		
Reps		

Prone Plank

	Set 1	Set 2
Weight		
Reps		

Bridge–Double Leg

	Set 1	Set 2
Weight		
Reps		

Living Wellness Workout 2

First time (set) through: Warm up: Go through all of the exercises slowly, 15-20 repetitions each, with no resistance (no weight), 5-10 minutes. Second set: Perform the exercises one at a time, with resistance when appropriate, starting with one lower body exercise, one upper body exercise, and one core exercise with minimal rest in between. Perform all nine exercises and repeat as your fitness goals and time permit! Remember to drink water during your workout and stretch tight muscles.

Lower Body

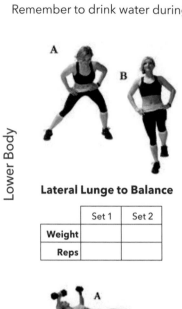

Lateral Lunge to Balance

	Set 1	Set 2
Weight		
Reps		

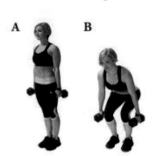

DB Squat

	Set 1	Set 2
Weight		
Reps		

SB Bridge–Double Leg

	Set 1	Set 2
Weight		
Reps		

Upper Body

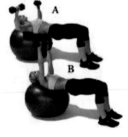

DB SB Chest Press

	Set 1	Set 2
Weight		
Reps		

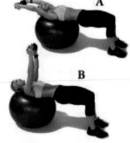

DB SB Lat Extension

	Set 1	Set 2
Weight		
Reps		

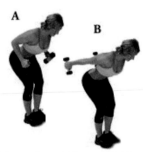

DB Bent Over Triceps Kickback

	Set 1	Set 2
Weight		
Reps		

Core

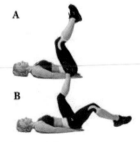

Scissor Kick–Bent Legs

	Set 1	Set 2
Weight		
Reps		

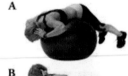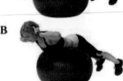

SB Back Extension

	Set 1	Set 2
Weight		
Reps		

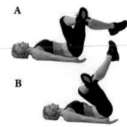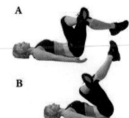

Cross-Leg Reverse Crunch

	Set 1	Set 2
Weight		
Reps		

Living Wellness Workout 3

First time (set) through: Warm up: Go through all of the exercises slowly, 15-20 repetitions each, with no resistance (no weight), 5-10 minutes. Second set: Perform the exercises one at a time, with resistance when appropriate, starting with one lower body exercise, one upper body exercise, and one core exercise with minimal rest in between. Perform all nine exercises and repeat as your fitness goals and time permit! Remember to drink water during your workout and stretch tight muscles!

Lower Body

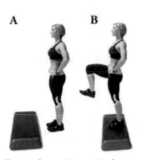

Front Step-Up to Balance

	Set 1	Set 2
Weight		
Reps		

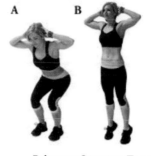

Prisoner Squat to Toes

	Set 1	Set 2
Weight		
Reps		

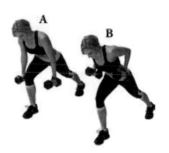

DB Lunge with Row

	Set 1	Set 2
Weight		
Reps		

Upper Body

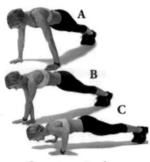

Crossover Pushup

	Set 1	Set 2
Weight		
Reps		

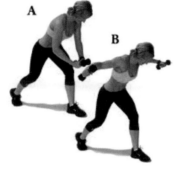

DB Lunge Reverse Fly

	Set 1	Set 2
Weight		
Reps		

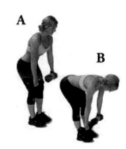

DB Deadlift

	Set 1	Set 2
Weight		
Reps		

Core

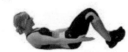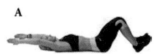

Pilates Half Roll Up

	Set 1	Set 2
Weight		
Reps		

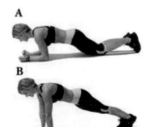

Knees Plank to Pushup

	Set 1	Set 2
Weight		
Reps		

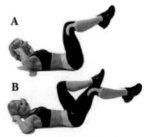

Supine Bicycle

	Set 1	Set 2
Weight		
Reps		

Living Wellness Workout 4

First time (set) through: Warm up: Go through all of the exercises slowly, 15-20 repetitions each, with no resistance (no weight), 5-10 minutes. Second set: Perform the exercises one at a time, with resistance when appropriate, starting with one lower body exercise, one upper body exercise, and one core exercise with minimal rest in between. Perform all nine exercises and then repeat as your fitness goals and time permit! Tempo: Count to four as you contract (tighten) your muscles during an exercise (exhale); release the exercise on a count of one (inhale). For example, count to four as you lower into a squat and count to one as you stand up. Remember to drink water during your workout and stretch tight muscles.

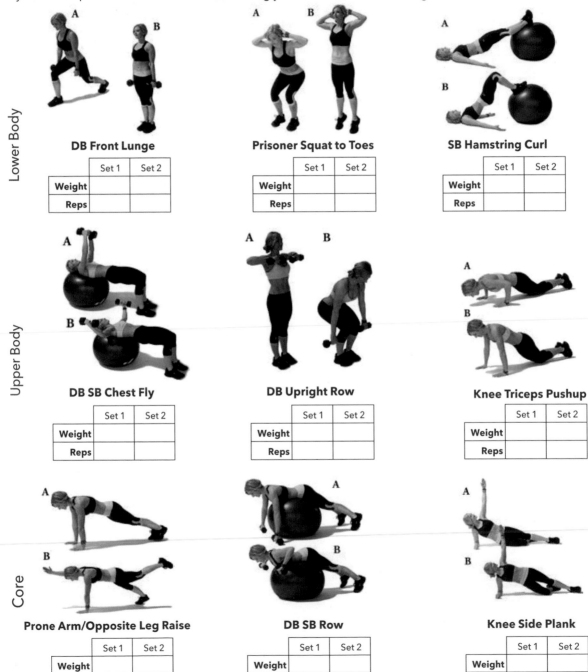

Lower Body

DB Front Lunge

	Set 1	Set 2
Weight		
Reps		

Prisoner Squat to Toes

	Set 1	Set 2
Weight		
Reps		

SB Hamstring Curl

	Set 1	Set 2
Weight		
Reps		

Upper Body

DB SB Chest Fly

	Set 1	Set 2
Weight		
Reps		

DB Upright Row

	Set 1	Set 2
Weight		
Reps		

Knee Triceps Pushup

	Set 1	Set 2
Weight		
Reps		

Core

Prone Arm/Opposite Leg Raise

	Set 1	Set 2
Weight		
Reps		

DB SB Row

	Set 1	Set 2
Weight		
Reps		

Knee Side Plank

	Set 1	Set 2
Weight		
Reps		

Stretching and Foam Rolling

Please allow time for foam rolling (self-myofascial release) and stretching! Flexibility is vital for injury prevention and muscle, joint, and bone health. According to the National Academy of Sports Medicine, research suggests that you can stretch before and after your workout. Stretching before you work out is *not* stretching cold muscles, as previously thought by fitness professionals. Light, static (holding, never bouncing) stretches and foam rolling before you begin may enhance your workout by eliminating tightness in muscles and allowing for a full range of motion during your workout. *Please refer back to this page after each workout for a full range of foam roll and stretching exercises.* If you do not have time to perform all the stretches, select stretching exercises that coincide with the muscles you just exercised and muscles that are tight. Hold each stretch for at least 30 seconds or 5-7 full breaths.

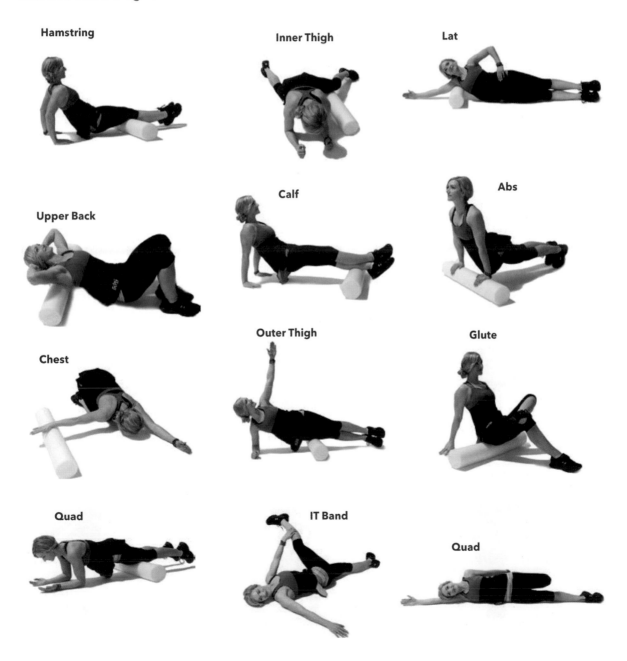

Hamstring

Inner Thigh

Lat

Upper Back

Calf

Abs

Chest

Outer Thigh

Glute

Quad

IT Band

Quad

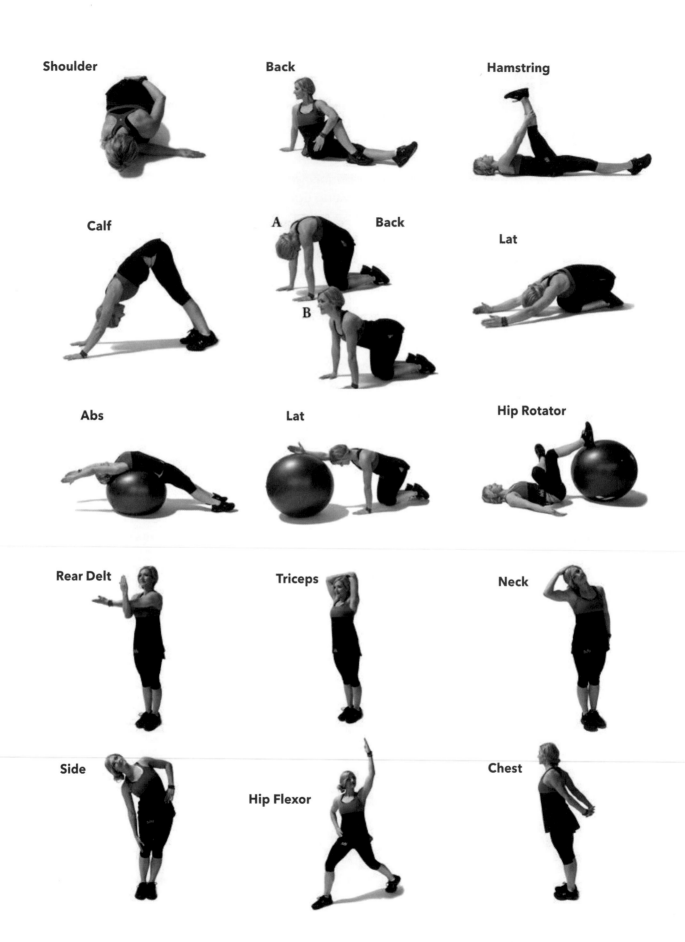

Shoulder

Back

Hamstring

Calf

A   Back

Lat

B

Abs

Lat

Hip Rotator

Rear Delt

Triceps

Neck

Side

Hip Flexor

Chest

Appendix M

Activity	Calories/30 minutes (180 lb. person)
Basketball	339
Bowling	57
Cycling (10 MPH)	246
Dancing (aerobic)	333
Dancing (social)	126
Gardening	225
Golf (pull/carry clubs)	210
Golf (power cart)	96
Hiking	201
Running slowly	417
Running	510
Skating (ice and roller)	264
Skiing (cross country)	339
Skiing (water and downhill)	255
Swimming (crawl, moderate pace)	348
Tennis	267
Walking	291
Weight Training	294

Notes

Week 1

American Cancer Society. "Normal Weight Ranges: Body Mass Index (BMI)." Information and Resources for Cancer: Breast, Colon, Lung, Prostate, Skin. 2013. Accessed March 19, 2013.

"American Heart Association Recommendations for Physical Activity in Adults." American Heart Association Recommendations for Physical Activity in Adults. Accessed June 17, 2016. http://www.heart.org/HEARTORG/HealthyLiving/PhysicalActivity/FitnessBasics/American-Heart-Association-Recommendations-for-Physical-Activity-in-Adults_UCM_307976_Article.jsp.

Anand, Preetha, Ajaikumar B. Kunnumakkara, Chitra Sundaram, Kuzhuvelil B. Harikumar, Sheeja T. Tharakan, Oiki S. Lai, Bokyung Sung, and Bharat B. Aggarwal. "Cancer Is a Preventable Disease That Requires Major Lifestyle Changes." *Pharm Res Pharmaceutical Research* 25, no. 9 (2008): 2200. doi:10.1007/s11095-008-9690-4.

Beard, Eric, Erin McGill, and Scott Ramsdell. *NASM Live: Essentials of Personal Fitness Training*. National Academy of Sports Medicine, 2011.

Borg, Gunnar. *Borg's Perceived Exertion and Pain Scales*. Champaign, IL: Human Kinetics, 1998.

Clark, Micheal, Scott Lucett, and Donald T. Kirkendall. *NASM's Essentials of Sports Performance Training*. Philadelphia, PA: Wolters Kluwer/Lippincott Williams & Wilkins, 2010.

Colbert, Don. *The Seven Pillars of Health*. Lake Mary, FL: Siloam, 2007.

Compart, Pamela J., and Dana Godbout Laake. *The Kid-Friendly ADHD & Autism Cookbook: The Ultimate Guide to the Gluten-Free, Casein-Free Diet*. Beverly, MA: Fair Winds, 2009.

Diederich, F. Remy. *Healing the Hurts of Your Past: A Guide to Overcoming the Pain of Shame*. Place of Publication Not Identified: Cross Point Publishing, 2006.

Eberle, Harold R. *Christianity Unshackled: Are You a Truth Seeker?* Shippensburg, PA: Destiny Image, 2009.

Epstein, Lawrence, and Steven Mardon. *The Harvard Medical School Guide to a Good Night's Sleep*. New York, NY: McGraw-Hill, 2007.

"EWG's Shopper's Guide to Pesticides in Produce." EWG's 2016 Shopper's Guide to Pesticides in Produce. Accessed June 17, 2016. https://www.ewg.org/foodnews/.

Harvard School of Public Health. "Artificial Colors." 2009. Accessed March 19, 2013.

Mayo Clinic. "Trans Fat Is Double Trouble for Your Heart Health." 2011. Accessed March 19, 2013.

Michaels, Jillian, and Mariska van Aalst. *Master Your Metabolism: The 3 Diet Secrets to Naturally Balancing Your Hormones for a Hot and Healthy Body!* New York, NY: Crown, 2009.

Office of Dietary Supplements. "Vitamin E." Dietary Supplement Fact Sheets. Accessed April 1, 2013.

Powers, Scott K., and Edward T. Howley. *Exercise Physiology: Theory and Application to Fitness and Performance*. Boston, MA: McGraw-Hill, 2009.

Prochaska, James O., John C. Norcross, and Carlo C. DiClemente. *Changing for Good: The Revolutionary Program That Explains the Six Stages of Change and Teaches You How to Free Yourself from Bad Habits*. New York: W. Morrow, 1994.

Rubin, Jordan. *The Maker's Diet for Weight Loss*. Lake Mary, FL: Siloam, 2009.

Silvoso, Ed. *Anointed for Business*. Ventura, VA: Regal, 2002.

TerKeurst, Lysa. *Made to Crave: Satisfying Your Deepest Desire with God, Not Food*. Grand Rapids, MI: Zondervan, 2010.

United States Department of Health and Human Services. "Get Enough Sleep." 2008. Accessed April 10, 2013.

United States Food and Drug Administration. "A Food Labeling Guide: Chapter 5. Ingredients List." 2008. Accessed April 10, 2013.

Week 2

Balch, Phyllis A. *Prescription for Nutritional Healing*. New York, NY: Avery, 2000.

Boschmann, M. "Water-Induced Thermogenesis." *Journal of Clinical Endocrinology & Metabolism*, no. 88.12 (2003): 6015-019.

Brennan, Georgeanne. *Salad of the Day: 365 Recipes for Every Day of the Year*. San Francisco, CA: Weldon Owen, 2012.

"Diet and Attention Deficit Hyperactivity Disorder - Harvard Health." Harvard Health. Accessed June 10, 2016. http://www.health.harvard.edu/newsletter_article/Diet-and-attention-deficit-hyperactivity-disorder.

Food and Nutrition Board. "Dietary Reference Intakes for Energy, Carbohydrate, Fiber, Fat, Fatty Acids, Cholesterol, Protein, and Amino Acids." 2005.

Havala, S. "Vegetarian Diets." *Journal of the American Dietetic Association*, no. 93.11 (2003): 748-65.

"How Much Sleep Is Enough?" - NHLBI, NIH. Accessed June 17, 2016. http://www.nhlbi.nih.gov/health/health-topics/topics/sdd/howmuch.

Johnson, Duke. *The Optimal Health Revolution: How Inflammation Is the Root Cause of the Biggest Killers, How the Cutting-Edge Science of Nutrigenomics Can Transform Your Long-Term Health*. Dallas, TX: BenBella, 2009.

APPENDIX & RESOURCES

Kidd, Kristine, and Kate Sears. *Weeknight Fresh and Fast: Simple Healthy Meals for Every Night of the Week*. San Francisco, CA: Weldon Owen, 2011.

Mayo Clinic Staff. "Metabolism and Weight Loss: How You Burn Calories." Healthy Lifestyle: Weight Loss. September 19, 2014. Accessed June 13, 2016. http://www.mayoclinic.org/healthy-lifestyle/weight-loss/in-depth/metabolism/art-20046508.

McCann D, et al. "Food Additives and Hyperactive Behaviour in 3-Year-Old and 8/9-Year-Old Children in the Community: A Randomised, Double-Blinded, Placebo-Controlled Trial," *Lancet* (Nov. 3, 2007): Vol. 370, No. 9598, pp. 1560–67.

"MSG Updates Introduction - Weston A Price." Weston A Price. 2000. Accessed June 17, 2016. http://www.westonaprice.org/health-topics/msg-updates-introduction/.

Powers, Scott K., and Edward T. Howley. *Exercise Physiology: Theory and Application to Fitness and Performance*. Boston, MA: McGraw-Hill, 2009.

Stella, George. "Vegetable Stir-fry." Food Network - Easy Recipes, Healthy Eating Ideas and Chef Recipe Videos. Accessed April 1, 2013.

Stokes, Tammy. *Your Healthiest Life: Mind, Body & Soul*. Charleston, SC: Advantage, 2010.

Stolze, Klaus, and Hans Nohl. "Free Radical Formation and Erythrocyte Membrane Alterations during MetHb Formation Induced by the BHA Metabolite, Tert -butylhydroquinone." *Free Radical Research* 30, no. 4 (1999): 295-303. doi:10.1080/10715769900300321.

"Sugar-Free Blues: Everything You Wanted to Know About Artificial Sweeteners - Weston A Price." Weston A Price. 2004. Accessed June 17, 2016. http://www.westonaprice.org/health-topics/sugar-free-blues-everything-you-wanted-to-know-about-artificial-sweeteners/.

"Trans Fat Is Double Trouble for Your Heart Health." Trans Fat: Avoid This Cholesterol Double Whammy. Accessed June 17, 2016. http://www.mayoclinic.org/trans-fat/art-20046114.

United States Department of Agriculture. "Trans Fats on the Nutrition Label." Food and Nutrition Services. Accessed August 19, 2013.

United States Department of Agriculture. "Center for Nutrition Policy and Promotion." 2010. Accessed August 19, 2013.

"What You Eat Can Fuel or Cool Inflammation, a Key Driver of Heart Disease, Diabetes, and Other Chronic Conditions - Harvard Health." Harvard Health. February 2007. Accessed June 14, 2016. http://www.health.harvard.edu/family-health-guide/what-you-eat-can-fuel-or-cool-inflammation-a-key-driver-of-heart-disease-diabetes-and-other-chronic-conditions.

Week 3

The American Heritage Dictionary of the English Language, Fifth Edition. Fifth ed. Houghton Mifflin Harcourt, 2011.

Ansel, Karen. "Is Gluten Bad for You." *Women's Health Magazine*, December 2010. Accessed April 5, 2013.

Compart, Pamela J., and Dana Godbout Laake. *The Kid-Friendly ADHD & Autism Cookbook: The Ultimate Guide to the Gluten-Free, Casein-Free Diet*. Beverly, MA: Fair Winds, 2009.

Deaths: Final data for 2013. National Vital Statistics Report. 2015;64(2). Detailed tables released ahead of full report: http://www.cdc.gov/nchs/data/nvsr/nvsr64/nvsr64_02.pdf[PDF-1.6M]. Accessed on June 3, 2016.

"Sprouted Grain." Food For Life. Accessed April 1, 2013. http://www.foodforlife.com.

Johnson, R. K., L. J. Appel, M. Brands, B. V. Howard, M. Lefevre, R. H. Lustig, F. Sacks, L. M. Steffen, and J. Wylie-Rosett. "Dietary Sugars Intake and Cardiovascular Health: A Scientific Statement From the American Heart Association." *American Heart Association*, no. 120.11 (2009): 1011-020.

Jonas, Wayne B. *Mosby's Dictionary of Complementary and Alternative Medicine*. St. Louis, MO: Mosby, 2005.

Nieh, Edward H., Gillian A. Matthews, Stephen A. Allsop, Kara N. Presbrey, Christopher A. Leppla, Romy Wichmann, Rachael Neve, Craig P. Wildes, and Kay M. Tye. "Decoding Neural Circuits That Control Compulsive Sucrose Seeking." *Cell* 160, no. 3 (2015): 528-41. doi:10.1016/j.cell.2015.01.003.

"Sugar-Free Blues: Everything You Wanted to Know About Artificial Sweeteners - Weston A Price." Weston A Price. 2004. Accessed June 17, 2016. http://www.westonaprice.org/health-topics/sugar-free-blues-everything-you-wanted-to-know-about-artificial-sweeteners/.

United States Department of Health and Human Services. "Carbohydrates." Dietary Guidelines for Americans. 2005. Accessed April 5, 2013.

Week 4

Bowden, Jonny. *The 150 Healthiest Foods on Earth: The Surprising, Unbiased Truth About What You Should Eat and Why*. Gloucester, MA: Fair Winds, 2007.

Compart, Pamela J., and Dana Godbout Laake. *The Kid-Friendly ADHD & Autism Cookbook: The Ultimate Guide to the Gluten-Free, Casein-Free Diet*. Beverly, MA: Fair Winds, 2009.

"Dietary Reference Intakes for Energy, Carbohydrate, Fiber, Fat, Fatty Acids, Cholesterol, Protein, and Amino Acids." Dietary Reference Intakes. 2005. Accessed April 1, 2013.

Erasmus, Udo. *Fats That Heal Fats That Kill*. Burnaby, BC: Alive, 1993.

Harvard School of Public Health. "Trans Fats." Harvard School of Public Health. 2009. Accessed March 19, 2013.

Johnson, Duke. *The Optimal Health Revolution: How Inflammation Is the Root Cause of the Biggest Killers, How the Cutting-Edge Science of Nutrigenomics Can Transform Your Long-Term Health*. Dallas, TX: BenBella, 2009.

Joseph, James A., Daniel Nadeau, and Anne Underwood. *The Color Code: A Revolutionary Eating Plan for Optimum Health*. New York, NY: Hyperion, 2002.

"Trans Fat Is Double Trouble for Your Heart Health." Trans Fat: Avoid This Cholesterol Double Whammy. Accessed June 17, 2016. http://www.mayoclinic.org/trans-fat/art-20046114.

United States Department of Agriculture. "Trans Fats on the Nutrition Label." Food and Nutrition Services. Accessed August 19, 2013.

Week 5

Balch, Phyllis A. *Prescription for Nutritional Healing*. New York, NY: Avery, 2000.

Bloom, Sophie. "What Are the Dangers of Synthetic Vitamins?" LIVESTRONG.COM. July 13, 2010. Accessed April 5, 2013.

"Bean Beef Burger." Healthy Cooking. March 31, 2010. Accessed April 5, 2013.

Conova, Susan. "Estrogen-Induced Cancer." *Estrogen-Induced Cancer*. Columbia University Health Sciences, n.d. Web. 09 Aug. 2016.

Holick, M. F. "Sunlight and Vitamin D for Bone Health and Prevention of Autoimmune Diseases, Cancers, and Cardiovascular Disease." *American Journal of Clinical Nutrition*, December 2004, 80.

Johnson, Duke. *The Optimal Health Revolution: How Inflammation Is the Root Cause of the Biggest Killers, How the Cutting-Edge Science of Nutrigenomics Can Transform Your Long-Term Health*. Dallas, TX: BenBella, 2009.

Krishnan, S., L. Rosenberg, M. Singer, F. B. Hu, L. Djousse, L. A. Cupples, and J. R. Palmer. "Glycemic Index, Glycemic Load, and Cereal Fiber Intake and Risk of Type 2 Diabetes in US Black Women." *Archives of Internal Medicine*, no. 167.21 (2007): 2304-309.

Mayo Clinic Staff. "Dietary Fiber: Essential for a Healthy Diet." Mayo Clinic. Mayo Foundation for Medical Education and Research. November 17, 2012. Accessed March 19, 2013.

Mellen, P., T. Walsh, and D. Herrington. "Whole Grain Intake and Cardiovascular Disease: A Meta-analysis." *Nutrition, Metabolism and Cardiovascular Diseases*, no. 18.4 (2008): 26.

National Osteoporosis Foundation. "Are You at Risk." Accessed April 5, 2013.

Pereira, M. "Dietary Fiber and Risk of Coronary Heart Disease." *ACC Current Journal Review*, no. 13.5 (2004): 26.

United States Department of Health and Human Services. "What Is Osteoarthritis." National Institute of Arthritis and Musculoskeletal and Skin Diseases. November 2010. Accessed August 19, 2013. HHS.gov.

Week 6

Abdelkafi, Sofia. "8 Homemade Vitamin Water Recipes." Sofia Abdelkafi Registered Dietitian. Accessed April 12, 2013.

American Heart Association. "Shaking the Salt Habit." April 22, 2013. Accessed March 5, 2013.

Balch, Phyllis A. *Prescription for Nutritional Healing*. New York, NY: Avery, 2000.

Bowden, Jonny. *The Most Effective Natural Cures on Earth: The Surprising, Unbiased Truth about What Treatments Work and Why*. Beverly, MA: Fair Winds, 2008.

Carlos, Juan. "Scientists Link Excess Sugar to Cancer." *Medical Research Journal*, February 2013.

"Just Give Me the FACTS!" Cereal FACTS - Home. Yale University. 2009. Accessed April 12, 2013.

Compart, Pamela J., and Dana Godbout Laake. *The Kid-Friendly ADHD & Autism Cookbook: The Ultimate Guide to the Gluten-Free, Casein-Free Diet*. Beverly, MA: Fair Winds, 2009.

Costenbader, Carol W. *The Big Book of Preserving the Harvest*. North Adams, MA: Storey, 2002.

"Sodium and Chloride." Dietary Reference Intakes. USDA Food and Nutrition Information. Accessed April 1, 2013.

Johnson, R. K., L. J. Appel, M. Brands, B. V. Howard, M. Lefevre, R. H. Lustig, F. Sacks, L. M. Steffen, and J. Wylie-Rosett. "Dietary Sugars Intake and Cardiovascular Health: A Scientific Statement From the American Heart Association." *American Heart Association*, no. 120.11 (2009): 1011-020.

Katz, Sandor Ellix. *Wild Fermentation: The Flavor, Nutrition, and Craft of Live-culture Foods*. White River Junction, VT: Chelsea Green Pub., 2003.

Katz, Sandor. "Making Sauerkraut." Wild Fermentation. April 27, 2012. Accessed April 19, 2013.

Mayo Clinic Staff. "Added Sugar: Don't Get Sabotaged by Sweeteners." Mayo Clinic. Mayo Foundation for Medical Education and Research. October 5, 2012. Accessed April 5, 2013.

McMillen, S. I. *None of These Diseases*. Westwood, NJ: F. H. Revell, 2000.

Michaels, Jillian, and Mariska van Aalst. *Master Your Metabolism: The 3 Diet Secrets to Naturally Balancing Your Hormones for a Hot and Healthy Body!* New York, NY: Crown, 2009.

"Release 25." Nutrient Data Products and Services. Accessed April 12, 2013.

Queen's University. "Chemists Shed Light on Health Benefits of Garlic." *Science Daily*, January 2009.

Seidenberg, Casey. "Fermented Foods Bubble with Healthful Benefits." *The Washington Post*, November 20, 2012. Accessed April 19, 2013.

Skorecki, K., and D. Ausiello. "Disorders of Sodium and Water Homeostasis." In *Goldman's Cecil Medicine*, by Lee Goldman and Andrew I. Schafer. 24th ed. Philadelphia, PA: Elsevier Saunders, 2011.

TerKeurst, Lysa. *Made to Crave: Satisfying Your Deepest Desire with God, Not Food*. Grand Rapids, MI: Zondervan, 2010.

United States Department of Health and Human Services. "Dietary Guidelines for Americans." Accessed April 5, 2013. Health.gov.

Week 7

Reall, Scott. *Journey to Freedom: Your Start to a Lifetime of Hope, Health, and Happiness*. Nashville: Thomas Nelson, 2008.

Week 8

Batterson, Mark. *The Circle Maker: Praying Circles around Your Biggest Dreams and Greatest Fears*. Grand Rapids, MI: Zondervan, 2011.

Dunbar, Brian. "Frequently Asked Questions." NASA. Kennedy Space Center. May 1, 2013. Accessed April 19, 2013.

Acknowledgments

God is holy. I am full of joy! Thank you, God, for the gift of voice and relationships. Thank you for the gift of your one and only son, Jesus, who I love more each day!

Writing a book is a little like raising children; it takes a village. I am so thankful for the village that helped and supported me with *Living Wellness for Growth Groups*. People are what make life's journey fun and exciting and worth living to the fullest. There are too many people to list here, so to everyone who was a part of this project in prayer or deed that didn't get listed by name, my most sincere *thank-you*.

Thank you to my husband, Casey, for your unwavering confidence, patience, strength, and encouragement in everything I do. Casey, you are my best friend, and I love growing old(er) with you! My beautiful children, Isabella and Kane, who keep me thinking, laughing, and growing with them all day long. You are my treasures!

My family: Debra, Tony, Dave, Rosie, John, and Tony for your support and love; my three sisters Sara, Caitlyn, and Alexis, who hold fragrant petals of tenderness in my heart; Ryan, Emily, Brent, Lisa, Tracy, Billie, and Aaron, in whose incredible families I am an addition and who helped shape my life growing up. I love you.

Co-founder and contributor, Dawn Brommer, for leaving your corporate job and taking a leap of faith into the world of health and wellness with me! Dawn, you are a beautiful person inside and out, and it has been an honor to write and promote this project with you!

Living Wellness Journal contributor, friend, colleague, and my right side Julie Frandsen. We shared much homemade sourdough bread, soaked nuts, and coffee as we examined *every word* of this book. Thank you for your patience, creativity, and confidence in me and this project. You have been so vital in the success of this project and company!

My adored friend and mentor Tracy Shearer who always steers me in the right direction. You are the humblest person I know. Thank you for always keeping me focused on the people and things that matter the most. Thank you for your careful help editing and contemplating the contents of this book.

My bro-in-law Marc Hanson and your beautiful bride (my sister Caitlyn Hanson), thank you for hunkering down on the porch for hours and hours of thoughtful attention. Marc, you bring a guy's perspective to the table J—you are a valuable addition to the Living Wellness team.

My dear, beloved friends for believing in me, helping me, and keeping me balanced. Colleagues for your encouragement and insight. Thank you for your thoughtfulness.

Living Wellness Growth Group participants and personal training clients for being my true inspiration for this book.

Dear friend Christina Zaczkowski, who helped to paint the pages of the first *Living Wellness* book with rich color and vibrant depth. You pour your heart into everything you do; Bjorn Dixon for your admirable and thoughtful foreword, which offers hope for health that reaches far beyond the physical body. And for your careful and attentive eye on all the scriptural and spiritual health components of this book. You always encourage me to pursuit my God-given dreams. Thank you.

Business affiliates who walk alongside my mission for a healthier community. We are transforming our communities together.

Editors: Specifically my cherished aunt Catherine Long for your careful and detailed work, patience, and teaching in the original *Living Wellness* book; Tony Darkenwald for your sense of humor and tenderhearted correction; Hanna Kjeldbjerg and the whole team at Beaver's Pond Press for your expertise; Kim Hanauska, you are one of the most detailed people I know—thank you for the professional and personal work you have done in all my companies and especially this book; Sara and Chris Ensey for your attention to detail; loyal directors, colleagues, assistants, advisors, mentors, and friends Carmen Trainor, Shannon Immer, Kelley Suggs, Steve Fessler, Mana Moini, Lauren Wallerius, Annie Stafford, Schwabs, Fitches, Schoemers, Dixons, and so many others—this book would not be possible without you.

Artists: James Zaczkowski for creating the *Living Wellness* logo, website, and countless other beautiful works of art; Alicia Black for designing the original workout layouts and tediously editing every exercise move; Jay Monroe and Dan Pitts for designing the cover and interior layout of both *Living Wellness* books—you have the ability to take a concept and creatively bring it to life; original fitness photography by Jacki Vaughan, owner of Jacki V. Photography, and cosmetologist, Aarica Larson, owner of InsparationSalon.

And last but certainly not least, you, my readers, who I may not meet in person but who invest in themselves through this book, to seek something unique—you are worth more than mediocre; you are worth living an abundant life. Thank you for entrusting me with your health. I pray this book will be a blessing as you continue to live in wellness.

About Ashley

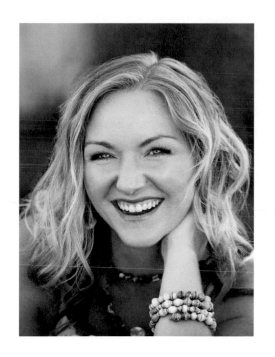

Ashley Darkenwald, MS, CPT, PES, loves pizza! And ice cream with peanut butter, and chocolate chip cookies. Years ago, Ashley realized that she was addicted to sugar and junk food nearly her whole life . . . and has paid the price with weight struggles, allergies, adult acne, and joint pain. Ashley started a journey to discover what it means to live a *balanced, abundant life* full of colorful nutrition, functional fitness, and deep spirituality. Ashley is passionate to share her health secrets with everyone! With more than ten years as a certified personal trainer and as an award-winning author, business owner, and mother of two, Ashley continues her journey of lifelong learning with her newest exciting book *Living Wellness for Growth Groups*!

"Christ is my destination.
Wellness is my passion. *Because we were created for more than mediocre.*"

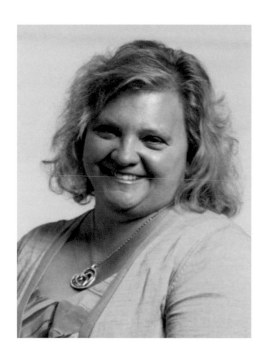

A note from Dawn Brommer,
co-founder of Living Wellness, LLC

When I was a little girl, I used to eat frosting under my bed when my dad abused my mom. As I got older, I drank diet coke to fill the void in my life. Nothing worked. It took me a while, but with the help of Living Wellness Growth Groups, I learned about what *truly nourishes* my body. I now fill the hole in my stomach with God's love, not unhealthy, sugary junk food.

My passion is to empower others
to make life-changing transformations.
Be blessed as you travel this journey!

The Conception of *Living Wellness for Growth Groups*

Oh, how life changes our dreams.

I received my undergraduate degree in political science, with an emphasis in pre-law. I wanted to be an ambassador traveling the globe and bringing about world peace.

Before college, however, I was a well-rounded athlete with an intense love of playing sports. I was a gymnast and a track-and-field athlete; my favorite event was pole vaulting.

While in college, I taught group exercise classes and worked at the student activity center. During this phase in life, I learned an important lesson that sports weren't just fun, they were also tremendously helpful in relieving stress. However, instead of turning to God *first* with my emotions, I turned to running. I ran when I was stressed. I ran when I was happy. I ran when I was sad. Unlike most of my college friends, I *lost* twenty pounds due to my obsessive running routine. I wanted to inspire others on their journey to health, so I became a personal trainer.

The first couple years of my training career were very successful. I implemented personal workout plans, and my clients were losing weight, getting stronger, reducing back pain, and feeling more confident. However, as time went on, the weight loss usually plateaued, and other physical issues tended to creep up. I was frustrated at the lack of long-term success.

It was around this time in 2007 that I took a nutrition course as part of my continuing education. I remember reading in one of the textbooks that long-term *weight loss is 80 percent nutrition and 20 percent fitness*. As a personal *fitness* trainer, this was a new concept to me. I started reading everything I could on nutrition, starting with publications from the Harvard School of Public Health, the Mayo Clinic, and the Centers for Disease Control and Prevention. My clients began implementing balanced nutritional practices, and results were fantastic. I confirmed that nutrition is a key aspect in weight loss. But I noticed something more when my clients cleaned up their nutrition: they experienced side effects of more energy, less chronic pain, fewer digestive issues, clearer skin, and fewer allergies. I also noticed all these side effects myself as I implemented better nutrition! The result was a dramatic improvement in the quality of our lives! I thought, *I have to share this knowledge with everyone*!

While I was researching and writing about fitness and nutrition, I had a life-changing experience with God. I remember the day clearly. I was out for a run when I believe God asked me the question, "*What are you doing with your life?*" I continued my conversation with God during the run and I came up with answers such as, "*I'm promoting the health and well-being of people*" and "*I'm improving the quality of life for my clients*." He asked me again, "*But why?*" I was struggling to answer this when I believe I clearly heard God say to me, "*I care about every cell, every detail, every part of your life, including your health, your body, and your emotional state. Do you care as much as I do? I have something better in mind for your life and your health. Will you receive the goodness I have for you?*" What?! I stopped running. God cares deeply about my physical health and well-being? At that time in my life, I was *not* taking good care of my emotional and physical health. I knew that God cared about my *spiritual* health. But I never gave much thought about all aspects of my health and faith being interconnected and equally important. I thought the body was just a temporary container for my spirit. During that encounter I felt convicted of how I had badly treated my body and mind, but I also felt deeply loved and cherished by God. I felt as though I had been struck by lightning, but had sustained no injuries.

This experience with God launched me into a hunger to see more of what God has to say about our physical and emotional wellness and to learn more about the character of God as a whole. It became very apparent that God cares for *all aspects* of his creation. This revelation put me on a path to seek out God's word regarding the connectedness of health in all aspects of life, which I believe is the definition of abundant life. This is where the Living Wellness journey began—connecting the knowledge of fitness and nutrition research with discovering God's desire for our lives.

The first *Living Wellness* book was published in 2014. The book is a fabulous read on nutrition education and foundational fitness information. It also includes a biblical affirmation in each chapter. Individuals and personal trainers use the book to gain a better understanding about how their bodies work and how to properly nourish their bodies rather than simply fuel them. Those who implement the practical knowledge in *Living Wellness* improve their quality of life. It's been beautiful to watch countless transformations.

In 2015, one particular client, Dawn Brommer, read *Living Wellness* and attended a series of my nutrition classes called "Are You Addicted to Sugar?" She instantly recognized that she and her family *were* addicted to sugar, and the consequences were evident. Reading *Living Wellness,* starting a consistent exercise routine, and attending the nutrition classes set Dawn on a journey toward mind, body, and spirit transformation. Dawn thought, *This book needs to be read within small groups everywhere!* She recognized the power of being able to talk through challenging concepts, ask questions, and give and receive encouragement in a group setting. After facilitating Dave Ramsey's "Financial Peace University" in a small-group setting, Dawn recognized that accountability was a major key in long-term success.

Dawn and I partnered up and made a plan for how to get the knowledge of *Living Wellness* delivered in a safe environment that promotes inspiration, mindfulness, accountability, and motivation. This plan takes into account the health of the whole person—mind, body, and spirit. With my expertise and experience in fitness and nutrition, the majority of this book's focus is physical health. However, as all aspects of your health are connected, you will have an opportunity each week to reflect and make action steps toward your mental/emotional and spiritual health.

We implemented beta groups to test out the small-group concept, and the results have spoken for themselves. Participants of the Living Wellness Growth Groups have lost weight, but the most significant changes have been seen in such comments as, "*I now eat to nourish my body, rather than eat to stuff myself,*" and "*I exercise out of respect for my body, rather than punishment,*" and "*It's so freeing to invite God into my health journey, I never thought to do that before.*" Participants of the Living Wellness Growth Groups are trusting God's promise for an abundant life, taking action toward that promise, and experiencing wholistic transformation of their minds, bodies, and spirits. Friends, get ready: it's *your* turn!

INDEX

smoothie recipes, 94

suggested serving size, 240

See also produce

G

garlic, 178–179

genetically engineered (GE) foods, 54

Gilmore, Dave, 202

GISSI Prevention Trial, 152

glucagon, 121

glutamine, using to reduce cravings, 115

gluten-free grains, 127

goals

brainstorming own, 19

components of, 17

God. *See* Jesus

grains

enriched, 74–75, 117–118

in FOSS chart, 52, 130, 236

gluten-free, 127

recommended servings per day of whole, 167

resources for information about, 243

soaked and sprouted, 127–129

Grilled Chicken with Pesto Sauce recipe, 230

Grilled Fish and Summer Squash recipe, 99

grocery shopping, 91–92

cost of produce, 100–101

label reading and, 72, 74, 126, 173

list for meal planning, 232–235

pesticide guide, 238

growth groups, described, 15

gut

balancing, 193

body health and, 192–193

fermented foods and, 194–195

H

habits, changing, 45–49

hamstring curl exercise, 204

Harvard School of Public Health, 151, 152, 176

Healing the Hurts of Your Past: A Guide to Overcoming the Pain of Shame (Diederich), 45

heart disease/attacks

omega-3s and, 151, 152

statistics, 119

sugar and processed food and, 119–120

heart rate zones, calculating, 25–26

Hippocrates, 170

homeostasis, 35

Hybels, Bill, 13, 51

hydrogenated fats, 148–149

I

inflammation

omega-3s to omega-6s balance, 155

types, 92–93

unprocessed foods and, 130

insoluble fiber, 166

inspiration, importance of, 16

insulin

dependency, 120, 121–122

response to unprocessed food, 130

International Journal of Chemistry, 178

iodine, 180

iron, food sources of, 56

INDEX

recommended servings per day, 167

sprouted grains instead, 128

wine, 195

women

body image and, 46

calcium and, 172

margarine and, 149

osteoarthritis risk, 170

osteoporosis risk, 170

workouts

1, 251

2, 252

3, 253

4, 254

guidelines for, 250

stretching and foam rolling, 255

See also cardio(vascular) training; exercises; strength training

Y

youth. *See* children

Z

Zaczkowski, Christina, 197

zinc, food sources of, 56

Reflection Notes:

Reflection Notes:

_____
_____
_____
_____
_____
_____
_____
_____
_____
_____
_____
_____
_____
_____
_____
_____
_____
_____
_____
_____
_____
_____

Reflection Notes: